Paediatric Surgery

MODERN PRACTICAL NURSING SERIES

This important new nursing series, designed specifically for the State Enrolled Nurse and Auxiliary Nurse is published as a 'parent' book covering the basic nursing skills entitled AN OUTLINE OF BASIC NURSING CARE, and a number of smaller handbooks covering the individual specialities as the nurse is moved from one discipline to another.

AN OUTLINE OF BASIC NURSING CARE: This aims to help the nurse learn the general basic nursing skills, and also how to apply them, and stimulate thought about nursing in differing hospital situations.

THE SPECIALITY BOOKS: Having mastered the basic nursing skills the pupil nurse will find herself attached to the nursing staff in any ward in the hospital. Although she is expected to play a part in this specialised ward team she may have had only a brief glimpse of the subject in her earlier training. It is for this stage in her career that this series of books is designed. The subjects covered include: Paediatric Orthopaedics, Theatre Routine, Paediatric Surgery, Dermatology, Urology, Adult Medicine, Geriatrics, Ear Nose and Throat, Mental Deficiency, Ophthalmology, Adult Orthopaedics, Plastics and Burns, Psychiatry, Obstetrics and Adult Surgery. All these are written by expert authors usually consisting of a doctor and sister tutor actively engaged in the work about which they have written and in touch with modern nursing trends.

These books are extensively illustrated and easy to use. As paperbacks they are inexpensive and it is hoped therefore that the nurse will have available a set of modern practical books which will help her in her ward work.

3

Modern Practical Nursing Series

Paediatric Surgery

Elizabeth D. Strathdee, R.G.N., R.S.C.N.
Ward Sister, Royal Hospital for Sick Children, Glasgow

Daniel Greer Young, M.B., Ch.B., F.R.C.S. (Edin.), D.T.M.&H.
Senior Lecturer in Paediatric Surgery,
The University Glasgow.
Honorary Consultant Surgeon,
Royal Hospital for Sick Children, Glasgow.

WILLIAM HEINEMANN MEDICAL BOOKS LIMITED: LONDON

This book is dedicated to the Matron and Nursing staff of the Royal Hospital for Sick Children, Yorkhill, Glasgow.

First Published 1971
© Elizabeth D. Strathdee and Daniel Greer Young
ISBN 0 433 31858 9

Printed by Redwood Press Limited,
Trowbridge & London.

Contents

1
Introduction

Paediatric surgery is that branch of surgery which is devoted to:-

a) The correction of congenital malformation such as cleft lip, cleft palate, oesophageal atresia, imperforate anus, urethral valves etc., and

b) The care of infants and children with surgical disorders. Conditions commonly dealt with in this group are hernia, intussusception, appendicitis, undescended testes.

The children's hospitals and the paediatric surgeons working in them usually deal with children up to about thirteen years of age. Thereafter the environment necessary in a children's hospital is no longer applicable to the teenage group and this latter group tend to be treated in adult wards. The children's hospital and nursing and medical staff working in them are orientated towards the specific problems of management and treatment of babies and children.

Progress in Paediatric Surgery

Progress in the surgical correction of congenital malformations has been more marked than the advances in any other branch of surgery in the last twenty years. Many factors have contributed to this. The essentials of pre-operative and post-operative care are better understood and surgery can now safely be considered for babies only an hour or two old and also for babies who are very small, e.g. under 2 kg. birth weight. The nursing staff play a vital role in the care of these very young patients and the paediatric surgeon is dependent upon close co-operation with the nursing staff who are in intimate contact with the babies. The nurse must report what might seem trivial details in an older child such as the baby not taking his feed satisfactorily or respiratory rate increasing a little over the previous few hours.

Apparently minor details like these pointed out to the surgeon may alert him that complications are developing.

Congenital Malformations

Most congenital malformations occur as a result of interruption in development or maldevelopment in the first three months of intra-uterine life. Few of the causes of these maldevelopments are known. In some such as cleft lip and cleft palate there is high familial incidence and genetic factors obviously play a part. However, genetic factors are not the sole determining reason for a baby developing a cleft lip or a cleft palate as environmental factors also have to interplay with these genetic factors. The means by which this interplay occurs is not known and in identical twins there is only a 1 : 4 chance of both infants having cleft lip or cleft palate. In other cases, infection of the mother with a virus such as the Rubella virus (German measles) may be the cause of a development anomaly such as congenital heart disease. That drugs administered to the mother in early pregnancy can cause maldevelopment of the foetus gained world-wide publicity with the tragic Thalidomide which caused multiple limb deformities. Unfortunately, thousands were affected before this drug was withdrawn in 1961 in Europe. Some other drugs are also known to have adverse effects on the developing foetus in the early weeks of gestation. Apart from genetic, infective and drug factors the other reasons for development of congenital malformations are not known.

Parents of Infants with Malformations

In treating an infant or child with a malformation it is very important to consider the parents and the entire family situation. With the birth of a baby with a congenital anomaly the parents often have a feeling that this is the result of something they have done, or that it is the result of some basic defect in them which has become apparent in the child's disability. Considerable time must be spent explaining to the

2

parents what is known of the disorder and in re-assuring them. No matter how clearly the explanation is given to the parents it is seldom that they can comprehend and accept what is told and patience must be exercised in reiterating the details on more than one occasion. It is also important to give the parents advice on the likelihood or otherwise of the defect presenting again in subsequent children they may have. Having achieved good rapport with the parents subsequent treatment of the child is more easy and with the parent's help, the co-operation of the child is usually much easier to obtain particularly if he is a toddler or young child.

The Newborn Baby and Surgery

Contrary to popular belief a newborn baby is not a bad surgical risk but withstands major surgery very well. In the neonatal period the baby will be apparently much less upset by a major chest or abdominal operation than a baby during the next few months of life when major operations are rather less well tolerated. This is in part due to the baby having an immature immune defence mechanism. In the first few days of life sufficient is carried over from the mother but over the next few months the baby's own immune defence mechanism is just developing. It is fortunate that many major surgical procedures may be necessary in the immediate period after birth but it is seldom that major surgery need be performed in babies a few months old and most can be delayed until they are larger and can withstand operation better.

Infants and Adults

Infants and children are not simply miniature adults and it is important to realise this in handling babies. The younger they are the more difference there is. If one considers the length of a baby at birth and the length of an adult it will be seen that the baby has to increase approximately three and a half times this length. If one looks at the baby's weight with an average British baby weighing 3.25 kg and the

3

adult 70 kg it will be seen that there has got to be a twenty times increase in the body weight. There is also a difference in body composition in that the newborn baby has a water content of 80 per cent whereas the adult has dropped to about 60 per cent.

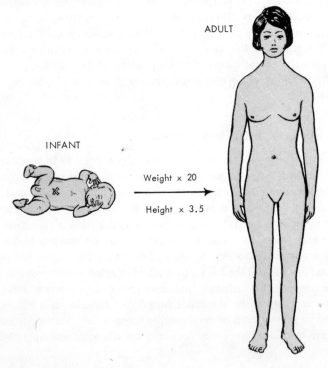

ADULT

INFANT

Weight × 20

Height × 3.5

Fig. 1.

Importance of Warmth

The newborn baby is also much less able to conserve heat and hence in nursing newborn babies great care must be taken to maintain body temperature. This is the reason for the ancient tradition of wrapping babies up in many layers of warm clothing. This fact must be kept in mind when a baby is exposed in the operating theatre or in the

4

ward for any procedures such as setting up an intravenous infusion. The environment must be kept warm for these small infants.

Heat production and heat loss are usually balanced so that a relatively constant body temperature is maintained. In newborn babies maintenance of body temperature is not so well stabilised and it is for this reason that they are nursed in a high environmental temperature which is most easily achieved by nursing them in incubators where the temperature can easily be regulated. The incubator is also useful for nursing infants after operation as they can easily be given increased oxygen when this is required but still can be freely observed for any abnormal signs.

Another feature of children is that it is dangerous to take the temperature in the mouth as the child may bite the thermometer and injure his mouth. It should be taken by either placing the thermometer under the axilla or in the rectum. For young infants a low registering thermometer should be used to prevent mistaken readings of 35.5-36°C when the baby's temperature may only be 32°C. When taking the temperature by rectum the thermometer is lubricated with K–Y jelly. The nurse should hold the child firmly to prevent him struggling and should hold the thermometer in position for one minute.

2
Hospital Admission

The Environment

The first impression most children have of hospitals is in their initial visit to Outpatients' Department or Casualty. The surroundings should be bright and with appointment systems practised in most hospitals waiting is reduced to a minimum. However, adequate play area and toys to occupy the children when waiting are necessary. Parents are allowed to remain with the child throughout the examination. All consulting rooms should be endowed with soft unbreakable toys and ideally the doctor present at the initial consultation should be present when the child is admitted to the ward. Children may become upset on admission through meeting so many strange and unfamiliar faces. Unlike outpatients' department, the casualty department deals with acute illness and traumatic injuries. The child is often frightened and upset and the parents, when present, are usually over-anxious for him. However, similar facilities should exist.

In case of accidents attempts should be made to have the parents of the unescorted child brought to him as soon as possible, thus relieving some of the child's anxiety. The flurried atmosphere which is often created calls for tolerance and understanding from the nursing staff who must appear calm throughout any emergency. All children are seen by the casualty doctor on duty and treatment given where indicated. No more than minor surgery should be performed in the casualty department.

Obvious features of a hospital ward designed for children are the smaller size of beds, cots, furnishings and instruments necessary on account of the small size of the patients. Precautions have to be taken to ensure that the environment is safe as children will pry into any corner. All hot pipes, radiators, stairways and elevators must be protected so that children cannot gain access to them and cupboards should, where possible, be out of children's reach. The ward temperature is maintained at 20°C as children, even when in bed asleep, are often exposed and require a high ambient temperature. With babies higher environmental temperatures are required as they can lose an excessive amount of heat from their large surface area.

A children's ward is rarely found to be quiet. Children generally seek the company of other children especially once they are recovering. This usually leads to the ward being noisy and there must be sufficient room for the children to be up and play. Ill children should be nursed away from those convalescing as they require more peace. Increasingly, mothers are accommodated with the child and for some this is important. When mothers are resident with children this requires some re-orientation of the nursing and medical staff as the mother, who is untrained to pick up early signs of alteration in the child's condition, then becomes the person in closest contact with the patient.

The recovery rate of children is usually much quicker and more complete than in adults. Sufficient toys and books should be provided and space allocated to allow the convalescing child to exercise his energy. Play therapists can help to keep the child occupied and it is essential that schooling should not be forgotten. If, following acute surgery, the school teacher in the wards starts the child off on lessons after a day or two this keeps the child occupied for part of the day. With chronic diseases this is even more important. Where possible a separate corner or room should be set aside for school. This allows ward routine to continue and allows the teacher and patients a chance to concentrate.

Admission Routine

Before admission to the ward the parents and child are seen by the ward doctor who takes a careful history and examines the patient. It is important to enquire about recent contact with infectious disease, as the child who has been in contact with infectious disease is not admitted except in emergency. If he must be admitted he is isolated, otherwise there is danger of widespread outbreak of the disease concerned. Important points in the history of the child should be double checked by the medical and nursing staff. The presence of any allergies to drugs or food which the child may have should be prominently recorded in the case notes. The child is fully examined by the doctor and then it is the turn of the ward nurse to see him. Initially the child's pulse, temperature and respiration are recorded and he is taken to the bathroom where he is given a warm bath 38-40°C. His mother may be allowed to accompany him to bath him. While the child is stripped opportunity is taken to examine him thoroughly including a careful inspection of the head for any evidence of lice. If these are found he is immediately treated with Suleo or some similar preparation. The nurse also has a close look at his skin again to exclude any infective condition such as scabies which may not have been picked up earlier. The height and weight are recorded. A waterproof identity band is secured around the child's wrist or, with a baby, to the ankle as these tend to slip off the wrist in small babies. This band should have the name, age or date of birth and hospital number on it. The child is then dressed in clean night attire and children of four years and under are put in a cot, while the older child is taken to bed. The child's clothing is parcelled up and returned to the parents. It is common practice to have the parents check these and sign that they have received them. The parents should be told what is to be done to the child and signed permission is obtained from them for the anaesthetic and operative procedures which are necessary.

If the child is not for immediate operation he should be allowed up. He can wear his dressing gown which should be easily accessible by his bedside. By letting the child up to move around and talk to other children he will quickly make acquaintances and settle.

If the child is admitted as an emergency and is very ill it will not be possible to bath him in this fashion and he is put to bed and given a bedbath if time permits. If he is going very quickly for operation then this will not be performed and he is simply dressed in a theatre gown and put to bed after he is weighed. The weight is necessary for estimating blood volume and for correct dosage of medicine. It is important for the nurse to check when the child last had something to eat or drink as this is very important to the anaesthetist. All children must have their identity band applied at the time of admission whether emergency or routine.

Before allowing the child's parents to go home the nurse admitting the child must check with the ward sister that all necessary information has been obtained and that the parents' telephone number (if they have one) is recorded. The parents are advised about visiting and when to contact hospital for further information.

Adults can understand the reasons for hospitalisation but it is more difficult for a child to accept being taken from the family to unfamiliar surroundings. To minimise this disturbance hospital routine should follow the pattern of family life as much as possible. Also, parents should be honest with their child and explain to him that he has to stay in hospital until he is well again. Many children are now more aware of hospital life from watching television programmes and it is common to see children playing at hospitals. If the parents take a sensible attitude to admission of the child it is rare for the child to be upset by hospitalisation. 'Free' visiting, already accepted in many children's hospitals is becoming the general pattern. Parents can come and go freely and can be of assistance to the overworked nurse. In some hospitals there are also facilities for the child's mother to come in and stay with him and this is of particular value where an infant who is being breast fed has to be admitted. It is also of value for some families where separation of the child would have an adverse affect. The resident mother, and to a lesser extent, the free visiting system requires alteration in the approach of nursing and surgical staffs. Whereas in the past the nurse was in the closest contact with the patient as the nursing staff did everything for him throughout the twenty four hours, many of the small chores in caring for the child are done by the resident mother. Mothers are not well trained to pick up early signs of disease hence greater vigilance on the part of the nursing and surgical staff is necessary or complications can develop and only be recognised at a relatively late time.

Investigations

There are a number of investigations frequently performed on infants and children and it is important that the nurse should know the routine for these. The commonly performed procedures are:-

Midstream Specimen of Urine

1   A trolley is cleaned and a sterile dressing pack is opened and laid out on it (see wound dressing, Page 24). This has:-
    a) Drapes
    b) Gallipots (2)
    c) Swabs
    d) Foil Bowl
    e) Forceps
2   Hibitane in water and saline should be placed in the gallipots.
3   A universal container for the urine specimen.
4   Laboratory forms and labels to apply to the container, on each of which the name, hospital number etc. are clearly inserted.

5 A clean bed pan or urine bottle.
6 A receptacle for the soiled swabs is pinned to the side of the trolley.

Procedure:

1 Wash hands thoroughly.
2 Place a drape under the patient's buttocks.
3 Swab the perineal area with hibitane from above downwards, cleaning the penis and foreskin in the male, and vulva and labia in the female.
4 Repeat swabbing with normal saline.
5 The male child then micturates into the bottle and the female into the bed pan.
6 When a good flow of urine is established the foil bowl is slipped in below the child to collect some urine and micurition is then allowed to continue into the bottle or bed pan.
7 Part of the urine is transfered to the sterile universal container which is sealed, labelled and sent at once to the laboratory with the forms.
8 The remainder of the urine is retained for 'ward testing' by the doctor.

Catheterisation

It may not be possible to obtain a midstream specimen or in some special circumstances it may be necessary to catheterise the bladder or an ileal loop when the child has had a urinary diversion. To prepare for this:-

1 Nurse washes her hands thoroughly and dries them.
2 A trolley is washed with hibitane and dried with a paper towel.
3 A dressing pack is opened on to the top of the trolley.
4 Forceps are opened and placed on the trolley.
5 A suitable sterile catheter is placed on the trolley.
6 Sterile K—Y jelly—small sample of some expressed from a larger tube on to a swab.

7 Universal container and forms as previously described.

8 Bags for disposal of instruments and dirty swabs are attached to the side of the trolley.

Procedure:

The procedure is explained to the child before commencing. Two nurses must be present and one restrains and re-assures the child if necessary. Nurse washes her hands thoroughly. The penile area or vulva is cleaned. A sterile drape is applied over the area. The catheter is lubricated with K—Y jelly. The foreskin is retracted or labia separated to expose the urethral oriface. The catheter is passed along the urethra to the bladder. The first few ml. of urine are discarded and samples then taken. If the catheter is to be left in it is strapped to the perineum and thigh. Either a spiggot is inserted into the catheter or catheter connected to a urinary collection sterile bag which is hung from the side of the bed. Females are usually catheterised by a nurse and males by a doctor.

Cystogram

This is performed as described for catheterisation. It is either done in X-ray Department or the child taken after catheterisation to the X-ray Department where radio-opaque fluid is run in to distend the bladder. The child is screened by the radiologist and films taken when the bladder is emptying.

Twentyfour Hour Collection of Urine

This may be requested for various reasons, e.g. for investigation into the presence of tumours, endocrine disorders or for assessment of renal function. Different preservative are necessary for the various tests and they are usually put into special two litre containers which are obtained from the laboratory. It is important that the bottles are not washed out in the ward and that all necessary particulars are correctly added to the label on the container, i.e. full name, age, hospital number, and the date and time of collection. Drug therapy is usually discontinued before commencement of the collection and where applicable all foodstuffs containing vanilla are best avoided.

In the young child who will not inform the nurse when urine is to be passed it is necessary to apply a urine bag or, in a male child, Paul's tubing may be strapped to the penis. These receptacles must be emptied hourly into the collection jar. A small catheter inserted into the urine bag is aspirated, or the Paul's tubing is emptied by freeing the knot on the end away from the penis.

Intravenous Pyelogram (IVP)

This is performed for diagnostic purposes to outline the collecting systems from kidneys, the ureters and bladder.

1 A trolley is laid as above and to the sterile dressing pack is added a 20 ml. syringe, needles of size the doctor requests, and hibitane in spirit to a gallipot. A file should be available to 'score' the ampoules.

2 Ampoules of Hypaque 45 per cent (20-30 ml.) in a bowl of warm water (38°C.)

The procedure is explained to the child and the nurse holds the child's arms as for a venepuncture. The doctor washes, transfers the Hypaque to the syringe and selects the appropriate needle. He introduces the needle into the vein and slowly injects the Hypaque. Close observation should be made of the child for any signs of shock or allergy, abdominal pain, palor, fainting, sweating or rigor. The procedure should immediately be stopped if these occur and adrenalin given if necessary. X-rays are taken at intervals after the injection.

Ventricular Tap

This is performed for diagnostic purposes or to relieve pressure on the ventricles. A dressing pack is laid on a clean trolley and the following added to it:-

Drapes.
10 and 20 ml. syringes.

Disposable lumbar puncture needle.
Manometer set if pressure is to be taken.
Hibitane in spirit (0.5%) to one gallipot.
Small quantity of collodion to second gallipot.

Bottom Shelf:

A razor for shaving the head.
Universal container
Laboratory forms
Airstrip dressing

Procedure:

This is performed by a doctor while the child is held firmly by nurse. After wrapping the baby in a blanket or sheet to restrain his arms he is held firmly with the head at the edge of the table. The older child may be anaesthetised before the ventricular tap is done.

The fontanelle area of the head is shaved carefully. Nurse must observe the baby's colour throughout the procedure and report any untoward effect. The needle is inserted into the ventricle. When the pressure and sample have been obtained a swab dipped in the collodion is held around the needle as it is withdrawn from the scalp to seal the puncture wound.

The cerebro-spinal fluid withdrawn, correctly labelled and dated, should be sent immediately to the laboratory. Where an air ventriculogram is to be performed the above procedure is performed and 30-40 ml. of cerebrospinal fluid aspirated slowly and 10 ml. less of air injected before withdrawing the needle.

Blood Culture

Numerous tests can be performed on blood and apart from the simpler tests like haemoglobin and electrolytes which may be estimated from a capillary sample taken from the finger or heel stab, a sample of venous blood is withdrawn by using a syringe and needle. In cases such as pyrexia of unknown origin, it is necessary to obtain specimens of blood for culture and these must be obtained under aseptic techniques. The doctor and nurse wear face masks.

A trolley is mopped with hibitane (0.5%) in spirit and dried using a paper towel. A small dressing pack is opened and to it is added:

> Sterile hand towel.
> 20 ml. syringe.
> Needles.
> Hibitane in spirit to a gallipot.

Bottom Shelf:

> Blood culture bottles, labelled with the patients
>   details date and time.
> Laboratory forms.

The doctor washes his hands thoroughly, drying them on the sterile hand towel. The nurse holds the child firmly, to allow the doctor access to the arm, neck, or groin vein from which blood is to be taken.

The doctor prepares the skin by washing with the antiseptic solution and inserts the needle attached to the syringe into the vein. Blood is then withdrawn and, after cleaning the top of the blood culture bottles with antiseptic solution, half the blood is injected into each blood culture bottle.

The bottle, together with the form bearing child's name, ward number, date and time of collection and revelant particulars of illness are sent to the laboratory.

Stools

Any deviation from the normal should be reported immediately to a doctor or nurse-in-charge. This may be blood or mucus in the stool, loose watery stools, or foul-smelling bulky stools. The stool should be kept for the doctor to see and do any tests he wishes.

When obtaining a specimen of stool for the laboratory it is usually only a small specimen which is necessary, not the whole of the motion passed. The specimen is put in a container, must be clearly labelled and sent to the laboratory with accompanying form. If instead of looking for infection in this stool, the doctor wishes the entire stools in the twenty four hours or over some days to go to the laboratory, it is necessary in the younger child to place a sheet of polythene inside the napkin as this stool can easily be collected from this smooth surface and the chemical requests necessary done.

3
General Care ✳

The nursing of surgical paediatric patients requires the same attention to patients' physical comfort as for any other age group. Except in the unconscious child, less attention to skin care is required than for instance an elderly patient after operation. However, these details remain important in paediatrics and if forgotten nasty pressure sores etc. can occur due to inexpert nursing. General features in care are considered in this chapter and special care necessary with specific disorders is dealt with subsequently.

Administration of Medicines

Medicines (drugs) can be administered in various forms. It is important that all medicines to be given should be written onto a prescription chart by the doctor ordering them. The medicine should be clearly written giving the date, time, method of administration and signed by the doctor. The nurse must always check she is giving the correct dosage of the medicine and, where necessary, two nurses must check the procedure. The medicine trolley should always be kept beside the nurse when doing the medicine round, to prevent children taking away any gaily coloured bottles which may catch their eye.

Routes of Administration

a) By Mouth:
When giving children medicine by mouth it is important

that the nurse checks that it is swallowed. Most manufacturers use syrup bases to make the medicine palatable. Some children have difficulty in swallowing tablets but they can, however, be crushed between two spoons and mixed in rose hip syrup or milk and can then be swallowed easily. Unless the medicine has to be given at specific times it is best for the child that he gets it after meals. Medicine should not be added in the baby's milk feed. A small drink should be given. Staining of the teeth by medicine can be prevented by the child sucking the medicine through a straw.

b) Intramuscular Injection

The needle is introduced well into the muscles of the thigh, the upper outer aspect of the thigh being the site preferred. Two nurses are necessary for this procedure as the child must be held firmly

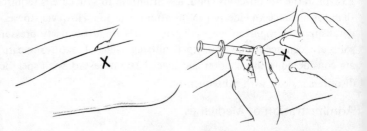

Fig. 3a Site of Injection   Fig. 3b Giving an Injection

to prevent a misplaced injection which can cause permanent nerve damage.

If given superficially the drug may cause fibrosis of the tissue or may result in abscess formation. The injection should be given alternately into the left and right thigh and as soon as possible the drug should be changed to an oral preparation. No more than 2 ml. should be given in one injection to a child and no more than 1 ml. to a small baby.

c) Intravenous Injection

The drug is given into the vein and the procedure carried out by a doctor.

d) Rectal Administration of Drugs

Drugs can be administered rectally in various preparations mainly by suppositories, pessaries, or retention enemata. For insertion of suppository or pessary it is necessary to have a small tray containing:

> Lubricant
> Prescribed suppository or pessary
> Finger cot or glove
> Swabs
> Disposal bag

The procedure is explained to the child and the bed screened. The child is placed on his left side with the right knee flexed over the left, and the hips flexed fully. The nurse puts on the finger cot or glove, lubricates the suppository or pessary and inserts it as far into the rectum as possible. The anus is cleaned with the swab and the glove disposed of. The child is then left quietly for ten minutes before being offered a bedpan, or the buttocks may be strapped together if the pessary is for retention.

Before giving some drugs rectally it may be necessary to wash out the bowel.

Articles required include:-

> Rectal catheter (20-24 F.G. tube).
> Tubing and connector.
> Funnel.
> Swabs.
> Lubricant, e.g. K–Y jelly.
> Warm normal saline (38°C).
> Polythene sheeting.
> Bedpan or container for return wash.

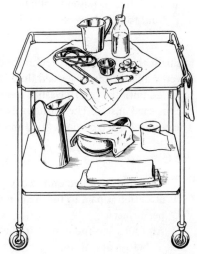

Fig. 4. Trolley.

The procedure should be explained to the child and requires two nurses. The child is placed on the left side and the upper part of the

17

body covered with a blanket. The lubricated catheter inserted well into the rectum. Fifty to 100 ml. of saline are placed in the funnel and by

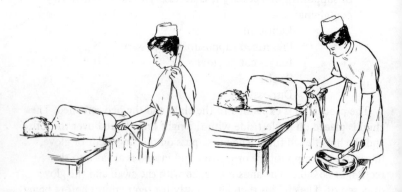

Fig. 5a Funnel is raised to allow fluid to flow into rectum.

Fig. 5b Syphoning back of faecal stained fluid.

raising it this runs into the rectum and colon. The funnel is then lowered and the faecal stained fluid is syphoned back. The procedure is repeated until the return wash is clear but should be stopped if the child becomes exhausted. The washout may be repeated daily until clear. The perineal area is cleaned, dried and the child returned to a warm bed.

Pre-Operative Care

1 The child is bathed on the day prior to operation and particular attention is paid to the area on which operation is to be performed.
2 All foods and fluids are with-held for a minimum of four hours before operation.
3 The infant or child who is vomiting has a naso-gastric tube passed and the stomach content aspirated. The tube is drained into a bag or small receptacle. It should not be blocked off as this would prevent it draining the stomach.

4 The anaesthetist orders premedication which consists of Atropine for the very young patients but for the older children over one to two years a sedative is given as well. This allays their apprehension while the Atropine or Hyoscine decreases the oral and bronchial secretions, and blocks potentially harmful effects which anaesthetic drugs given later might produce. Premedication is given from half to one hour before operation according to the instruction of the anaesthetist.

5 All babies undergoing operation in the first week of life are given Vitamin K 1mgm. on admission.

6 The identification bracelet is re-checked to ensure that the details are correct.

7 The child is then changed into a theatre gown and allowed to settle.

8 All relevant notes and X-rays of the patient are gathered so that they may be taken to theatre with him.

9 Results of any tests done in the hour or two immediately before operation should be obtained and written down for the surgeon and anaesthetist to see.

10 Where blood for transfusion has been requested a check is made that it is available and correctly labelled.

11 Occasionally a child will require intravenous fluids pre-operatively. This is usually to counteract dehydration induced by vomiting. Preparation for setting up intravenous infusion

a) Clean and mop the surface of a trolley with hibitane (0.5%) in spirit.

b) Open dressing pack.

c) Open dressing forceps on to the sterile pack.

d) Pour antiseptic solution, e.g. hibitane (0.5%) in spirit, into gallipot.

e) Open intravenous infusion set. For infants a special type of drip set which has a small graduated chamber holding 30 to 100 mls. of fluid is used so that an accurate knowledge of the volume of fluid given can be recorded.

f) The intravenous needle, intracath and scalp vein needle should be placed on the under shelf of the trolley so that whichever the doctor requests is available.

g) Intravenous fluid, as requested, is obtained and a bottle holder applied so that it may be hung on an infusion stand. A wide variety of fluids are available for intravenous therapy and so it is necessary to ascertain which fluid is required.

h) If no attachment is present on the incubator or bed for hanging up intravenous fluids an infusion stand is obtained.

i) Adhesive strapping and the appropriate size of splints e.g. for a baby two wooden spatulae stuck together and suitably padded, or for an older child a formal splint, are placed on the trolley undershelf.

j) The intravenous giving set is connected to the bottle. The bottle is then suspended from the infusion stand and fluid is run through the infusion set until all air bubbles are removed from the tubing. It is then ready for connection to the needle or cannula after this is introduced into the vein.

12 If the infant or child has no vein into which a needle can be inserted, the alternative method is to give intravenous fluids by a 'cut-down'' on a vein. This is usually on an ankle or elbow vein but any accessible vein will do. The area is anaesthetised and the catheter is passed into the exposed vein and ligated in this position. The skin wound is then resutured. To prepare for this:-

a) Trolley with a dressing set is laid out as previously described.

b) The cut-down set containing scalpel, fine-toothed and non-toothed dissecting forceps, artery forceps, retractors, needle holders, plain catgut, atraumatic silk sutures, is opened and placed on the dressing trolley.

c) To this is added antiseptic solution for cleaning skin, a 2 ml. syringe with needles (a larger one for aspirating, a fine one for injection), intravenous cannula of size selected by the doctor, local anaesthetic, e.g. Xylocaine 1 per cent, and an 'airstrip' dressing to cover the wound.

d) Splint and strapping for fixing the limb is prepared and applied either immediately before or after cut-down. This limb is lightly splinted to protect the intravenous infusion and is usually lightly tied to the side of the bed or cot to prevent the child moving it excessively and possibly displacing the drip.

e) Intravenous infusion set is set up as previously described ready to be connected to the cannula when it is inserted.

13 When the infant or child is called to the theatre he is taken in his incubator, cot or bed, or he may be transfered to a trolley if the former is not possible. His notes, charts and X-rays should go with the accompanying nurse. For the infant or child requiring intravenous infusion the chart of all fluid intake and output is also taken. This aspect is more fully considered in Post-operative Care. (Page 22).

Operative Care

Before the child is taken to the theatre it is essential to have the necessary equipment prepared. The theatre nurse sets up instruments in theatre while another nurse or theatre orderly checks the anaesthetic room. If an emergency arises it more often does during induction of anaesthesia and usually does so very quickly, hence everything must be ready to cope with such an emergency. For instance, the child may vomit and he is then in danger of asphyxia from inhalation of vomit. There should be available:-

    a) A supply of oxygen
    b) Face mask
    c) Oral airway
    d) Laryngoscope
    e) Endotracheal tubes
    f) Suction apparatus which has been checked
    g) Suction catheters for pharynx and smaller one for trachea
    h) Syringe and needles
    i) Drugs—sodium bicarbonate, calcium gluconate or chloride, adrenalin, coramine
    j) Stomach tube
    k) Lubricating jelly (e.g. K—Y)

This apparatus must be checked to ensure that it is working satisfactorily. The anaesthetist also requires a supply of drugs and anaesthetic gases.

The child is then taken to the anaesthetic room or, in the case of neonates, they may be taken straight from their incubator to theatre thus minimising exposure. The child should be allowed to take his favourite 'cuddly' toy along with him as this tends to allay his apprehension, but with his sedative he should be quite drowsy. Anaesthesia is induced and whenever the child is asleep anything he has brought along with him may be laid aside. Once the child is safely anaesthetised the ward nurse can go.

The patient is then taken into theatre and placed on the operating table in the position required by the surgeon. The younger the child the more care must be taken to ensure that he is not unduly exposed as babies can lose heat excessively from their relatively large surface area. This loss of heat will result in a fall in body temperature. Neonates or small sick infants should be placed on a heated blanket and exposed as little as possible as only by doing this will they be kept at normal body temperature.

When diathermy is to be used careful application of the indifferent electrode or diathermy pad is essential. If there is inadequate contact between patient and the pad then serious diathermy burns can occur. The surgeon and anaesthetist should also check that the nurse has satisfactorily applied the pad. This pad can either be a lead plate covered completely by a saline-soaked cloth bag or dry aluminium foil is used. This latter method is more safe. The position of the anaesthetised patient must be carefully checked to ensure that there is no undue strain on any joint, and that there is no pressure on any nerves, as the unconscious child cannot move. There should be no undue friction between the patient and any appliance around him.

Post-Operative Care

At the end of operation the child is not returned to the ward until he has come out of his anaesthetic. With modern techniques this usually means keeping him in a recovery room for ten or fifteen minutes, but longer may be necessary. Until he has regained consciousness he must be watched continuously by a nurse to prevent dangerous complications occurring. The main point is to make sure that the patient maintains an adequate airway. Obstruction of the airway will give rise to a serious lack of oxygen which may either permanently damage the brain or may kill the child. Obstruction may be due to:-

a) The tongue falling back into the pharynx and blocking it. This is prevented by maintaining the patient in a semiprone position. He is placed lying on one side with the uppermost leg flexed at hip and knee. The jaw is maintained forward by gentle traction on the lower jaw so that the tongue does not slip back and obstruct the airway. At this stage the anaesthetist will usually have left an oral airway in and once the patient has recovered he will spit it out.

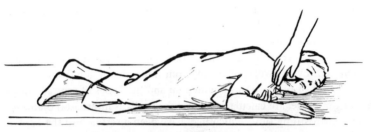

Fig. 6. The jaw is maintained forward by gentle traction.

b) By vomiting the patient may block his airway. Any child who has had an anaesthetic may vomit and he is in particular danger from this until fully conscious. The semi-conscious child has poor reflexes to prevent the vomit passing from the pharynx into the trachea. This is particularly likely to happen if the child is left lying on his back and is less likely to occur if he is maintained on his side. Vomiting also occurs very easily in small babies and is particularly dangerous in this group so great care is necessary.

While the patient is in theatre the incubator, cot or bed to which the patient has to be returned is prepared so that he returns to a warm environment. The patient who has recovered from an anaesthetic is still very sleepy and is initially nursed on his side as described in the immediate post-operative period. As the child wakens, he moves around

23

and usually spontaneously starts to sit up. The ill child will not sit up but should then be propped up as would an adult. Small infants are allowed to lie on one or other side and should be changed from side to side every two hours. This helps to prevent the development of pneumonia.

Oral feeding may be commenced four hours after general anaesthesia except when major surgery has been performed, or where operation has been on the abdominal cavity. Re-introduction of oral feeding is then delayed and may not be recommenced for twenty four hours or longer. Fluids are given first and then food is gradually re-introduced. A child with peritonitis from appendicitis may not be able to tolerate oral fluids for some days.

Where intravenous fluids have been commenced before or during operation they should be continued at the rate prescribed. Careful entry should be made on the fluid charts of all fluids given. On these charts all aspirate from naso-gastric tubes, urine produced etc. should be entered. Every twelve or twenty four hours the intake from oral, intravenous or other routes is added up and the losses of aspirate, urine and from bowel are calculated. Any tubes such as intercostal drainage tube, gastrostomy tube, which may have been inserted into the baby in theatre must be very carefully protected. The child's limbs must be restrained, e.g. by applying tube gauze over the hands and gently tying the limbs to the side of the cot. This is done particularly in the immediate post-operative period as the child recovering from an anaesthetic may be very restless and may try to pull out his tubes. Dislodgement of any of these tubes can be dangerous.

Most wounds are dressed in theatre and are left untouched until it is time to remove the sutures in five to ten days. However, other wounds such as infected wounds in the child with appendicitis and peritonitis or the child who has an abscess drained will require dressing. The procedure is:-

a) A trolley is prepared by cleaning with hibitane (0.5%) in spirit, opening a dressing pack on the top shelf, and adding dissecting forceps. On the bottom shelf hibitane lotion, adhesive tape, bandage, hand towel and spray of nobecutane or antibiotic powder are placed.

b) The patient is then brought to the treatment room.

c) Adhesive and superficial dressings are removed.

d) The nurse washes her hands thoroughly.

e) Sterile drapes are laid around the area to be treated giving a 'clean' area.

f) Using dissecting forceps the dressings remaining over the wound are removed and placed in the disposal bag, and these forceps are discarded.

g) The area is cleaned with hibitane soaked swabs.

h) The area is then dried with swabs again using dissecting forceps and not touching the area with the fingers.

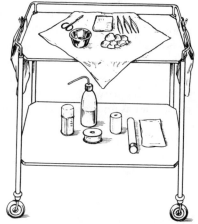

Fig. 7. A trolley is prepared.

i) A dressing is then applied. This may either be a swab placed over the wound and maintained in position by adhesive strapping.

Two variants of this procedure of wound dressing are dressing of wounds from which there is a purulent discharge, e.g. after drainage of an abscess and, secondly, dressing of a wound and removing sutures. For dressing a wound which has a purulent discharge the procedure described above is carried out down to item (f). If there is a drain into an abscess cavity, e.g. a piece of soft rubber or polythene, instructions may have been given to shorten this. To do this the drain is withdrawn from the wound a short distance and with a pair of sterile scissors the outermost part is cut off but leaving sufficient protruding from the wound so that the procedure can be repeated on subsequent days. A safety pin is inserted through the drain by using dissecting forceps. This prevents the drain from slipping through the wound into the abdominal cavity. A culture swab will be taken of the purulent material if the doctor requests this. It should be labelled with the patient's name and hospital number, and the date and time of when it was taken. The swab in its container and the laboratory form are sent to the bacteriological laboratories as soon as possible. If there is much discharge from the wound then in redressing the wound a large absorbent pad is applied and this is bandaged or strapped in position.

For removal of sutures a dressing trolley is set up in a similar fashion but added to it are forceps for holding the stitches and a pair of stitch scissors. These are sharp pointed scissors for insertion of one blade between the suture and the skin. The procedure is carried out as for dressing a wound until reaching the point (g).

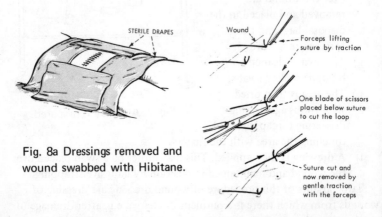

Fig. 8a Dressings removed and wound swabbed with Hibitane.

Fig. 8b Removing Sutures.

The sutures are then removed. This technique is simple but the child needs re-assurance that the approach of instruments is not going to result in pain. With each suture one of the long ends is held up and the point of the scissors is insinuated between the suture and the skin, the suture cut and gently pulled out. This procedure is repeated until all sutures are removed. The area is then cleaned again with hibitane and dried.

Post-operative complications of the respiratory tract are largely avoided by active mobilisation of the child in the early post-operative phase. Sometimes it is necessary to enlist the help of the physiotherapist to get the child's lungs fully re-expanded. In some special situations such as operations on the chest, physiotherapists are always involved in post-operative management in encouraging the patient to fully re-expand the lungs and cough up secretions.

Unlike adults, children are very much easier to manage post-operatively in that when they are fit they will get on the move and it will be extremely difficult to restrain them. However, they will not do themselves harm as, when they are tired or if a part is hurting, they will automatically return to their beds to rest the part of the body concerned. Hence a rigid routine for each individual child for every type of operation is not laid down and children will continue to surprise one in the rate at which they recover post-operatively.

4

Head and Neck

Mouth or Throat

Removal of the tonsils and adenoids is usually performed by the Ear Nose and Throat surgeons and will not be discussed. Operation for hydrocephalus is considered in Chapter 10. Operations on the head and neck are to excise cysts and fistulae, to correct deformities such as cleft lip and palate, to drain abscesses or to perform tracheostomy. Tracheostomy may be performed for a number of reasons, e.g. upper airway obstruction when tracheostomy is necessary to allow entry of air into the trachea and bronchi so that the child can breathe adequately, or because a baby is unable to cough up tracheo-bronchial secretions, or to enable the child to be connected to a ventilator for artificial ventilation for a prolonged period. Care of the tracheostomy is dealt with in Chapter 5.

Cysts and Fistulae

A variety of cysts and fistulae occur in the head and neck. These are excised and for this the child is admitted from the waiting list and has routine care.

Deformities

A number of 'plastic' procedures are performed on the head and neck, e.g. correction of bat ears. These children require routine nursing care and on return from theatre the corrected ear is protected by a dressing which is usually retained for two to three weeks. If the bandage is becoming loose it should be taken off and re-applied, leaving the dressing on the ear undisturbed.

Cleft Lip

This condition is obvious at birth. The defect may extend right up into the nostril, i.e. be a complete cleft lip or it may only extend part of the way to the nostril, i.e. incomplete cleft lip. The condition occurs in about 1 : 1,000 births and it is one of the congenital anomalies in which genetic factors play a part. It is approximately twice as common in the male as in the female and if one child has a cleft lip then the chance of a further child in the family having cleft lip drops from 1 : 1,000 to 1 : 30. Associated with cleft lip there may be a cleft palate but the two can occur independently.

A baby born with a cleft lip causes considerable distress to the parents. They have to be re-assured that this can be corrected surgically and it is often of value to show photographs of babies with cleft lip and following surgical repair. Operation is usually delayed until the baby is approximately three months although some surgeons may operate on the baby in the first two or three weeks of life. Until operation the baby has a dental plate fitted into which he sucks. This improves the alignment of the gums. He is fed either by using a teat with a large hole in it, or else by spoon feeding the baby. The mother can learn very rapidly to feed the baby by cup and spoon and this is done just before operation so that in the immediate post-operative period when the cup and spoon feeding is essential the baby can take feeds from a spoon.

Pre-Operative Care

Routine pre-operative care is given to the baby. Nasal and throat swabs are taken to ensure that there are no pathogenic bacteria which might cause infection of the wound. The infant's haemoglobin has to be checked.

Post-Operative Care

At the end of operation a Logan's bow is applied to the face. This is a metal bridge which is attached to the cheek by adhesive strapping. The purpose is to take tension from the upper lip and allow the lip to heal satisfactorily.

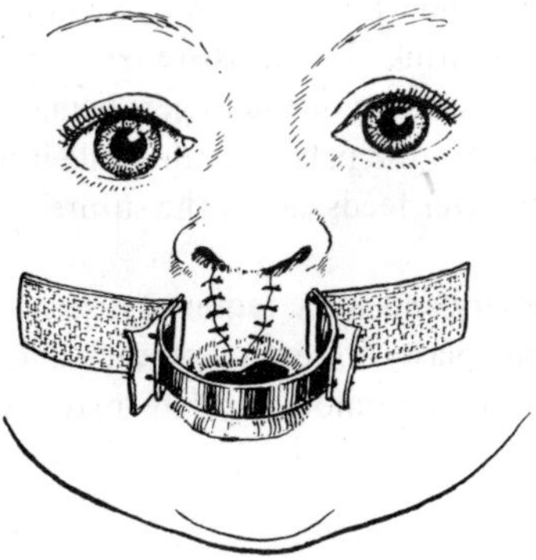

Fig. 9. Logan's Bow.

Post-operatively the infant has to be fed by cup and spoon and after each feed the baby's lip and mouth is cleaned. This is done by gently mopping the lip and nostril with saline soaked cotton wool and after cleaning off any crusting or scabbing, carefully drying the area. This has to be repeated with each feed. After seven days the sutures are removed from the upper lip and the Logan's bow remains until the tenth day. Throughout this period it is important to prevent the baby picking at the lip with fingers. To achieve this it is best to apply arm splints which prevent the baby flexing the elbows.

Cleft Palate

Cleft palate may accompany a cleft lip or may occur independently. Operation is usually performed at approximately fifteen months.

Pre-Operative Care

The infant is admitted two days before operation to check haemoglobin level, throat and nasal swabs for any organisms which may cause infection. Blood is cross-matched.

Post-Operative Care

It is important to ensure the infant's airway remains adequate in the twenty-four hours following operation. Some surgeons may leave a stitch in the tongue with long ends coming out of the mouth and strapped to the chin. If the airway is becoming obstructed gentle traction on this suture will pull the tongue forward to relievs the infant. The tongue stitch should not be removed until the surgeon says it is safe to do so. After each feed the infant's mouth is cleansed by giving him 30 ml. of sterile water or dextrose to drink. The arms are restrained as described in cleft lip to prevent thumb sucking or the fingers being inserted into the mouth and interfering with the palate repair while it is healing. Diet should be soft and a drink after feeds cleans the suture line.

Follow-up of these children is necessary and some require assistance from speech therapists or later, pharyngoplasty to improve speech and stop the 'nasal' speech which the short or immobile palate may result in.

Abscess

In infants and children abscesses in the neck are common. These usually arise in the submandibular or cervical lymph glands. Where pus has formed incision and putting a drain in the abscess cavity is necessary. The neck requires dressing at least once a day and the drain is shortened or removed when the surgeon feels the cavity is closing and the infection overcome.

5
Chest

The indications for chest operations in infants and children are usually a malformation which has occurred during development. Congenital heart disease is the commonest of these and it is not surprising that this complex double pump system does not always develop perfectly. Oesophageal atresia is the next most common anomaly requiring operation on the chest in infants while other conditions such as lobar ephysema are rare.

Congenital Heart Disease

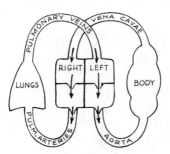

Fig. 10a.
Normal Circulation

The normal heart pumps blood from the left side to all parts of the body where oxygen and nutrients are taken up and waste products including carbon dioxide passed to the blood which returns to the right side of the heart. The right side pumps blood to the lungs where carbon dioxide is eliminated and oxygen taken up before blood comes to the left side of the heart for circulation to the body again. Defects in this system may make themselves apparent by the baby being cyanosed (bluish discolouration). This cyanosis which may be present very early in life is due to blood with insufficient oxygen being circulated to the body.

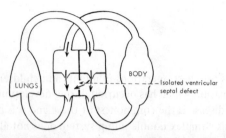

Fig. 10b. Cyanotic Congenital Heart Disease

In rather less serious malformations the cyanosis may be evident
on exertion and become more obvious as the child grows. The other
group of babies and children with congenital heart disease are acyanotic,
i.e. they do not have this bluish discolouration. An example of this is
the ventricular septal defect where there is an opening between the left
and right ventricles.

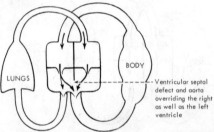

Fig. 10c. Acyanotic Congenital Heart Disease

Because the pressure in the left ventricle is higher blood flows from
left to right. This causes an excessive strain on the heart though survival
for months or years is not uncommon. These abnormalities are usually
detected on listening to the baby's heart and hearing a cardiac murmur.
Large defects may cause cardiac failure early in life.

Investigation of these children includes estimation of haemoglobin,
X-ray of chest, electro-cardiogram and, to define the precise defect, a
catheter is passed into the heart. Blood samples and pressures are taken
from various points and the child is X-rayed after injection of radio-
opaque material. By assessing the results of all these the precise defect
can be defined.

When cardiac failure supervenes the infant or child may be improved by supportive medical treatment with drugs such as digitalis and diuretics.

Operation is necessary to correct the anomalies. In some instances it is technically impossible to do this completely but in others the defect is so complex that correction cannot be achieved. New techniques of operation are being developed and even in infants function of the heart can be taken over for a time during operation, i.e. cardiac by-pass where blood is taken from the great veins, oxygenated and pumped into the aorta for circulation to the body again. This allows the surgeon time to correct the defect in the heart. With some congenital heart defects it is best to perform an operation in infancy which allows the baby to grow and develop and then some years later total correction of the anomaly can be achieved.

Pre-Operative Care

This consists of the normal routine care plus administration of drugs prescribed to ensure that the child's cardiovascular system is in the best possible state before operation. The child may also require physiotherapy to the chest pre-operatively to clear secretions from the lungs and decrease the risk of post-operative pulmonary infection and collapse.

Post-Operative Care

This varies with the extent of the surgical procedure and the size of the patient. Drugs and oxygen are given as prescribed and a frequent record of the pulse, heart rate, respiration and temperature are carefully charted. With more extensive surgery it may be necessary to give complex post-operative care with artificial ventilation by a machine through a naso-tracheal or tracheostomy tube and monitoring of the heart rate, blood pressure and frequent biochemical estimations on blood samples. In these complex cases a doctor should be supervising the patient continuously in the post-operative period. Routine nursing care of the child is given and careful records are maintained of the fluid intake and output. Care of intercostal drainage tubes and of intubated patients are dealt with below.

33

Intercostal Drain

After thoracotomy—where the chest wall and pleural cavity have been entered—a drainage tube is passed through a separate skin incision, between the ribs into the pleural cavity. This tube is sutured in position and when the chest wall is closed air may be trapped in the pleural cavity between the lung and the chest wall. This tube allows the air to drain out and must be connected to an underwater seal drainage bottle.

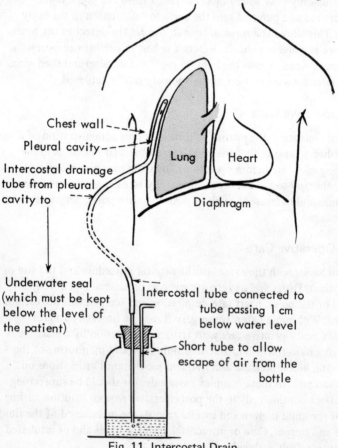

Chest wall - - -

Pleural cavity - - -

Lung   Heart

Intercostal drainage tube from pleural cavity to - - -

Diaphragm

Underwater seal (which must be kept below the level of the patient)

Intercostal tube connected to tube passing 1 cm below water level

Short tube to allow escape of air from the bottle

Fig. 11. Intercostal Drain.

It is important to check that the tube from the chest is connected to the bottle correctly, i.e. it must be connected to the glass rod which passes down under the level of the water by 1 cm. On inspiration fluid is sucked up this glass tube and on expiration the fluid level then falls. If the fluid level is not oscillating there is usually a kink in the tube which must be straightened. This bottle must always be kept below the level of the patient. It should *never* be raised above the level of the patient as fluid will then be syphoned into the chest. When moving the patient the tube should be clamped off to prevent any chance of fluid being syphoned into the chest or of air being allowed to escape up the tube back into the pleural cavity. When the tube is to be removed which is once the lung is fully expanded the suture holding the tube in position is cut and suction is applied to the tube as it is removed from the chest. A sterile swab is pressed over the opening in the chest wall as the tube is removed to prevent air leaking into the chest and a dressing applied over the small wound. For this the sterile dressings trolley is set up as for dressing a wound elsewhere.

Naso-Tracheal Intubation and Tracheostomy

With either of these procedures a tube is inserted into the trachea through the nose and pharynx, into the trachea in the former (Fig. 12a).

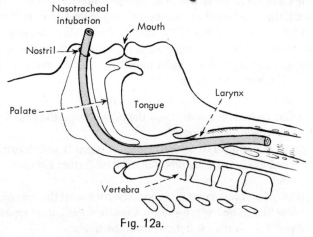

Fig. 12a.

and through an opening in the skin and subcutaneous tissues in the front of the neck in the latter. (Fig. 12b).

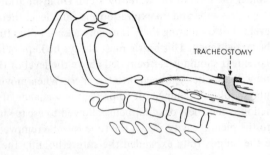

TRACHEOSTOMY

Fig. 12b.

Careful nursing is vital to the survival of these patients and a 'special' nurse is required for any patient with this. Aspiration of secretions from the lungs is necessary to prevent blocking of the tube and also to prevent retention of the secretions which will become infected. The tube is firmly strapped in position if it is a naso-tracheal tube or, with tracheostomy, the tube is tied around the baby's neck and must be securely fixed. The nurse must ensure that it remains so and that the child has a free airway. The patient is nursed with the neck extended, this is achieved by placing a small sandbag or a rolled up napkin below the shoulders. If the patient is not able to breathe adequately a ventilator is connected to the tube. Whether the patient is ventilated or not bronchial toilet must be performed every thirty minutes. The procedure for this is:—

1 ½ml. of saline is injected down the tube.
2 A fine catheter is passed down the tube beyond the end of it into the trachea and bronchi.
3 Suction is applied to this catheter as it is gently withdrawn.
4 Procedures 2 and 3 are repeated until no further aspirate is obtained.
5 It may be necessary to reconnect the patient to the ventilator and allow him to be oxygenated for a few minutes before repeating 2 and 3 to clear all secretions from the trachea.

36

Displacement of these tubes is very dangerous and danger signs are laboured breathing, restlessness, attempted phonation and cyanosis. Should any of these develop a doctor should be summoned at once.

When the tube is no longer needed it is simply removed and continued 'special' nursing of the patient is required in the succeeding twenty four hours to ensure that ventilatory problems do not supervene. The tracheostomy opening in the neck simply requires a sterile dressing applied over it and the opening usually closes very rapidly without any surgical intervention.

Oesophageal Atresia

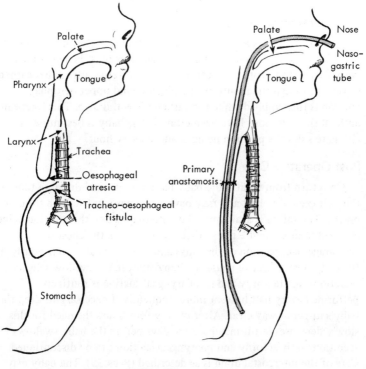

Fig. 13

This anomaly, where the upper oesophagus ends blindly, was

invariably fatal until the last thirty years. A high success rate is now achieved unless the baby has multiple anomalies. Associated with the oesophageal atresia there is usually a tracheo-oesophageal fistula and this abnormal communication between the lower oesophagus and the trachea must also be dealt with. These infants are often born after a pregnancy complicated by hydramnios and the baby at birth is 'mucusy'. Salivary secretions tend to dribble from the baby's mouth and there may be associated cyanotic or choking attacks dye to inhalation of these secretions. On attempting to pass a stomach tube it is held up by the atresia about 10 cm. from the lips. Diagnosis is confirmed by X-ray examination.

Pre-Operative Care

Routine care for a neonate is given and intermittent aspiration of the pharynx and proximal pouch of oesophagus must be performed every fifteen to twenty minutes. To do this a sterile soft rubber catheter is passed through the mouth to the pharynx and upper oesophagus. Suction is then applied while the catheter is withdrawn. This is repeated until all the secretions have been cleared. The baby is best nursed on alternate sides the position being changed every hour.

Post-Operative Care

On return from theatre the baby has an intercostal drainage tube through the right chest and may have a fine naso-gastric tube from one nostril. The infant is again nursed on alternate sides, the position being changed hourly. Gentle physiotherapy is given to the chest to encourage re-expansion of the lungs and this is repeated four hourly. In the early post-operative phase the baby still cannot swallow salivary secretions satisfactorily and so pharyngeal suction is routinely performed every half hour or more frequently if necessary to keep the baby's upper airway clear. After twenty four hours the need for this slowly decreases but it may be some days before the baby swallows secretions satisfactorily and pharyngeal suction can be discontinued. Care of the intercostal drain is as described (Page 35). The baby may have an intravenous infusion running post-operatively. Twenty four hours after operation feeding by the fine nasogastric tube may be commenced.

As this tube has a very small lumen feeds have to be injected down and this is best done by giving the baby small quanties hourly and then gradually increasing the feed volume and the time interval. One week after operation the baby can be tried with oral feeding and the initial oral feeds are of dextrose and then milk, once the baby has shown that swallowing is satisfactory. The stitches are removed from the chest wound after eight to ten days and once the baby is feeding satisfactorily he can be discharged home.

While the above is the standard treatment for a baby with oesophageal atresia the defect varies from one infant to another and a number of other procedures are sometimes necessary. These include oesophagostomy where the proximal oesophagus is brought out on to the neck, gastrostomy for feeding and this is described in the subsequent chapter. In these infants reconstruction of the alimentary tract may be done at a later stage by bringing the colon up to join with oesophagus above and oesophagus or stomach below.

6
Abdomen

Most operations on the abdominal cavity are on the alimentary tract and it is these which are considered in this chapter. The alimentary tract is in effect a tube extending from the mouth to the anus. Various parts of this tube have specialised functions: for instance, the stomach acts as a reservoir and this part of the tube is expanded so that a meal can be taken into it and then slowly passed into the duodenum and small bowel for further digestion and absorption of the nutrient materials. Undigested materials and some waste are passed along the bowel and through the anus. Indications for operations on the abdominal cavity are:—

1 Congenital anomalies of the alimentary tract, e.g. duodenal atresia
2 Infections, e.g. acute appendicitis
3 Obstruction (including intussusception)

4 Trauma, e.g. road traffic accidents
5 Tumours, e.g. neuroblastoma

1 Congenital Anomalies

One of the commoner causes of vomiting in infancy is *congenital hypertrophic pyloric stenosis.* This condition occurs between two and ten weeks of age and male infants are much more commonly affected than females. Vomiting is caused by the muscle surrounding the pylorus, i.e. the outlet from the stomach, becoming markedly hypertrophied and thickened so that this ring of muscle constricts the canal and blocks the outlet from the stomach. This thickened muscle is known as the pyloric tumour and the history of these infants is that they progress satisfactorily for the first week or two of life and then develop projectile vomiting, i.e. the vomit shoots from the baby's mouth and may land some distance from the baby. The vomit does not contain bile as the obstruction is above the level of the bile ducts entering the duodenum.
If vomiting is allowed to continue

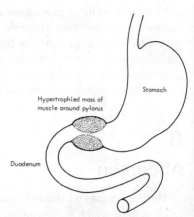

Fig. 14. Congenital Hypertrophic Pyloric Stenosis

the infant rapidly looses weight. Constipation is common. The diagnosis is made by giving the baby a 'test feed,' i.e. a normal milk feed is given and while the nurse is feeding the baby, the abdomen is inspected and palpated. Waves of visible peristalsis passing across the upper abdomen from left to right can be seen and the pyloric tumour is felt in the right subcostal region. Operation is then usually advised.

Atresia (complete loss of the lumen of the bowel) and *stenosis* (narrowing of the lumen) may occur at any level along the alimentary tract. It is most commonly found at the lower end of the alimentary tract (ano-rectal anomalies), in the duodenum, or in the small bowel.

Infants with imperforate anus should be diagnosed on routine post-natal examination but if missed then the infant presents in the next few days with abdominal distention, vomiting and failure to pass meconium.

Duodenal atresia is not visible externally. This causes vomiting within the first twenty four hours of life. The vomit is usually bile-stained and diagnosis is confirmed by X-ray examination of the abdomen. About one third of the babies with this anomaly are Mongols (Down's Syndrome) and half are under 2.5 kg. at birth. Small bowel atresia may occur in the jejunum or ileum and causes vomiting which usually commences within twenty four hours of birth but occasionally does not until the second or third day. The vomit is bile-stained and the baby's abdomen is distended. No meconium is passed and X-ray confirms the diagnosis. Meconium ileus is similar in presentation to ileal atresia but in this condition the infant has cystic fibrosis (fibrocystic disease of the pancreas) and the obstruction is due to the sticky secretions in the lumen of the bowel being so tenacious that they cannot be passed along the lumen. As well as operation to relieve the obstruction these infants require intensive and continuous therapy for their cystic fibrosis for the rest of their lives.

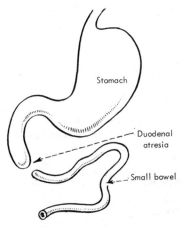

Fig. 15. Duodenal Atresia

2 Infections

Acute appendicitis is rare in the first year of life but thereafter becomes a relatively common disease. The infant or young child with acute appendicitis differs only in the fact by the time diagnosis is made there is usually spread of infection from the appendix to the peritoneal cavity, i.e. peritonitis. This occurs because the early signs and symptoms of appendicitis either are not present in the very young or are impossible to detect. The child of two does not localise pain well and so cannot tell when he has the early central abdominal pain which later settles down in the right iliac fossa. The child may just be generally unwell and have some vomiting and pass loose stools. Diagnosis is made on examination of the abdomen.

3 Obstruction (Including Intussusception)

Apart from the congenital causes of obstruction dealt with there are many causes of obstruction such as bands, herniae, volvulus etc. and these all cause abdominal pain and vomiting. Diagnosis is usually by X-ray of the abdomen and naso-gastric tube is passed and intravenous fluids are commenced pre-operatively. One peculiar form of abnormality occurring in infants particularly between the fourth month and the first year of life which progresses to obstruction is intussusception. This is where the bowel folds inside itself and causes severe colicky abdominal pain, vomiting and passage of blood and muscus per rectum. On examination of these infants the bowel folded

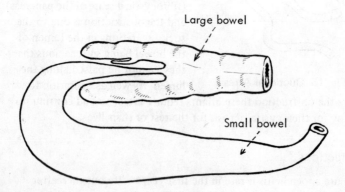

Fig. 16 Intussusception

in on itself can be felt as a sausage-shaped mass and X-ray examination may also be helpful in diagnosis.

4 Trauma

An increasing number of children are seen with multiple injuries from road traffic accidents. These frequently involve the orthopaedic and the general paediatric surgeon. Injuries to the liver, spleen, kidneys or gut may occur in these accidents and require urgent operation. Profuse blood loss, for instance, with a ruptured spleen occurs into the peritoneal cavity and urgent transfusion of blood is necessary to maintain an adequate circulation until operation is performed and the damaged spleen removed. Management of these children requires close team co-operation.

5 Tumours

Two of the commoner tumours arising in the abdominal cavity are the nephroblastoma arising in the kidney and the neuroblastoma which arises from the posterior abdominal wall often above the kidneys. The signs and symptoms are non-specific and the child is frequently just vaguely unwell. He may have some vomiting and diarrhoea and then the mass is palpated during routine examination of the abdomen. Surgical removal is the most efficient means of treating these tumours but full excision is not always possible and then the addition of cytotoxic drugs such as Actinomycin D, Vincristine and Cyclophosphamide and also treatment by radiotherapy can help. The outlook for children with neuroblastoma is very serious and the survial rate is still only around 20 per cent but with nephroblastoma it is 50 per cent.

Pre-Operative Care

The infant or child who is still vomiting should have a nasogastric tube passed pre-operatively. This tube must be of sufficient size to allow free drainage of the gastric contents and will vary depending on the size of the child. An 8 F.G. oesophageal tube is the smallest used for a neonate and for older children a larger tube. Nurse and an assistant should be present for passing the tube. The nostril area is cleaned. The tube is then taken from the packet and measured on the outside of the body, approximate length from the nose along the nasal floor to the pharynx and to the position of the stomach in the left upper quadrant of the abdomen. Having measured the length of the tube which requires to be passed a marker is placed on the tube, e.g. a small piece of adhesive on the tube. The tube is lubricated with KY jelly and passed over one nostril to the pharynx. At this level the child may retch but he is encouraged to swallow as the tube is advanced. Once in the stomach, gastric contents will be able to be aspirated easily. The tube is firmly strapped to the nostril but care must be taken to ensure that no pressure is being exerted on the edge of the nostrils as, with prolonged intubation, a pressure sore can occur. A syringe or suction machine is then attached to the tube and the stomach contents aspirated. Aspiration should be repeated hourly till operation and immediately before the child goes to theatre. Between aspirations the nasogastric tube should be allowed to drain freely into a bag. A careful record of the volume of gastric aspirate must be kept.

Intravenous fluids will be necessary for the dehydrated child and are set up as described (Chapter 3). A careful record of the volume of fluid infused and of the type of fluid given must be kept. Accurate fluid balance charts are kept recording all fluid given, and fluid loss by vomit, gastric aspirate, urine etc. Drugs prescribed by the doctor are given pre-operatively as is routine pre-operative care.

Post-Operative Care

Babies and children who have had laparotomy require particular attention because of the increase in the likelihood of these patients vomiting. If a nasogastric tube has been left in place following an operation it should be kept draining freely into a container at the patient's side. Every four hours the tube should be aspirated or the nasogastric tube may be connected to an intermittent suction to ensure the stomach is kept empty until the gut resumes peristalsis. Gastric aspiration must not be continued for long without intravenous replacement of fluid. When the gastric aspirate decreases oral feeding can be recommenced and the patient is gradually returned to normal feeds over a few days. With babies in particular it is common practice to start with a little dextrose in water then gradually to increase the quantities and strength of the milk feeds after the baby has shown that he is taking the feeds and not vomiting.

There are some special features of abdominal operations requiring nursing attention.

Gastrostomy (Fig. 17)

Gastrostomy is where an opening is made in the abdominal wall and a tube passed through this and into the stomach. The stomach is usually stitched to the anterior abdominal wall. This tube must be

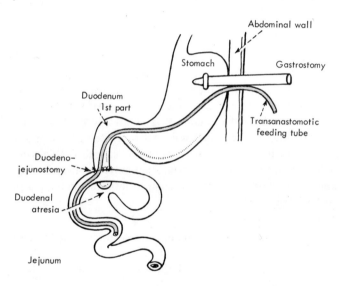

Fig. 17. Gastrostomy.

carefully retained in place particularly in the first week after operation. The tube is firmly strapped on to the anterior abdominal wall and to achieve maximum fixation it is best to paint the skin with some Friar's balsam after thoroughly cleaning it and drying it, and then to apply half inch adhesive tape around the tube and on to the abdominal wall in two separate directions. This tube may be kept draining into a receiver. It replaces the nasogastric tube. Once feeding is

recommenced the tube is either hung up on the side of the cot or
incubator with a funnel or syringe barrel into which feeds may be
poured. After a week the danger of changing the gastrostomy tube or
removing it is much less. If a tube is in for a long time a check must
be made regularly that the tube is not slipping further into the stomach
as it can be passed into the duodenum and cause obstruction. This is
done by gently pulling the gastrostomy tube back until resistance is
felt with the wings of the catheter pressing against the anterior
abdominal wall.

Ileostomy and Colostomy

Infants and children may require an ileostomy or a colostomy and
as with adults the care of the skin surrounding this is important. These
'ostomies' are frequently only temporary until a more major operation
is performed on the bowel when the baby is bigger. Some parents
find it easier to have the child with a colostomy discharge faeces
on to the anterior abdominal wall and to protect the skin around
the colostomy by painting it with Whitehead's varnish. A napkin is
applied around the child's abdomen. Alternatively colostomy bags may
be applied and this is done with the same routine as applying bags to an
ileostomy (Figs. 18, 19):-

1 Clean and dry the skin.
2 Paint the skin to the margin of the colostomy with Tinc. Benz.
    Co.
3 Apply the adhesive bag with the hole cut to the size of the
    colostomy over it, or
4 Dip a karaya gum washer and then apply this around the
    colostomy moulding it to the correct size.
5 A phlange is placed on the karaya gum and stuck in position with
    adhesive strapping.
6 A collecting bag is applied over the phlange.
7 Netaplast may be used as a sort of corsette and the length of
    Netaplast cut. An opening is cut in the middle of the band of
    Netaplast and this slipped over the child's abdomen. This helps
    to retain the bag in place.

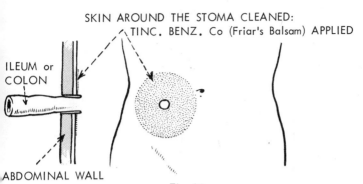

SKIN AROUND THE STOMA CLEANED:
TINC. BENZ. Co (Friar's Balsam) APPLIED

ILEUM or
COLON

ABDOMINAL WALL

Fig. 18a

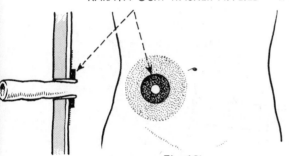

KARAYA GUM WASHER APPLIED - if desired.

Fig. 18b

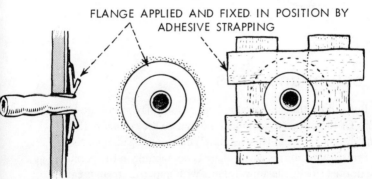

FLANGE APPLIED AND FIXED IN POSITION BY
ADHESIVE STRAPPING

Fig. 18c

47

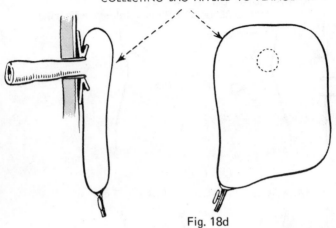

COLLECTING BAG APPLIED TO FLANGE

Fig. 18d

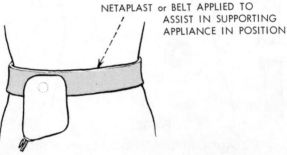

NETAPLAST or BELT APPLIED TO
ASSIST IN SUPPORTING
APPLIANCE IN POSITION

Fig. 19.

7
Rectum and Anus

Both congenital and acquired conditions may affect the rectum and anus. Of the congenital anomalies only two are common, the imperforate anus and Hirschsprung's disease or aganglionosis.

Imperforate anus is where there is no opening in the perineum at the normal site of the anus. Infants with imperforate anus can be grouped into one of two types. The first type is the imperforate anus with a low fistula, i.e. where there is an abnormal and usually small communication between rectum and the perineum. This opening is situated anterior to the site of the normal anal opening (Fig. 20a).

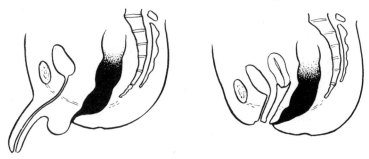

Fig. 20a Imperforate Anus—Low Fistula

The second type is where the rectum ends above the pelvic floor musculature and from the rectum a fistula runs forward into the urethra in the male or into the vagina in the female. This latter group of babies often have other anomalies as well as the ano-rectal anomaly. These other anomalies frequently affect either the urinary system or the cardio-vascular system. The diagnosis of imperforate anus should be made on routine post-natal examination. Operation is necessary for these babies.

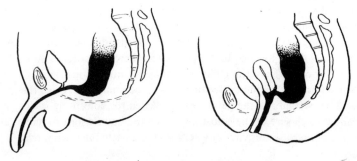

Fig. 20b Imperforate Anus—High Fistula

Pre-Operative Care

Pre-operative care is the routine care for a neonate undergoing operation. The operation performed depends on the anomaly present.

Post-Operative Care

Post-operative care of these infants is to commence dextrose feeds four hours after operation and then to introduce milk. To prevent stenosis or narrowing of the new anal opening daily dilatation by either a Hegar's dilator (No. 12 for an average sized infant) or by using the fifth finger is performed. Dilatation should be continued for two to three months to ensure that late stenosis does not occur. It is important to follow these babies in the first few months to ensure that the bowels are functioning satisfactorily. If this is done then long term results are good.

Colostomy is performed for the babies with a high fistula (Fig. 20b). Post-operative care is that of the colostomy and the gradual introduction of oral feeding twelve to twentyfour hours after operation.

Before the baby is discharged from hospital the distal loop of bowel from the colostomy down to the pelvis is given a washout. This is performed in similar fashion to a rectal washout using warm normal saline and when a clear washout is obtained the distal bowel has been emptied. The infant is then allowed home and some months later the child is re-admitted for a major operation which consists of a laparotomy, division of the fistula to the urethra or vagina and pulling the bowel down through to the perineum where it is stitched to the skin. Post-operatively the child continues on intravenous fluids for twentyfour hours and oral feeding is then recommenced. Once the child has settled and the perineum has healed the colostomy is closed. Following closure of the colostomy when the bowels start to move care of the perineal skin is vital or a very sore excoriated perineum may result.

The skin of the perineum is throughly cleaned when the nappie is changed after each feed. The area is dried and cream is applied. Zinc oxide cream may be sufficient or in other children Colibar or Tannafax applied to the perineum helps protect the skin. If the skin continues to be excoriated exposure of the buttocks and perineal area with the application of a mixture of egg white and brandy usually allows the area to heal. Thereafter nappies are re-applied once the area is thoroughly cleaned and cream applied.

Hirschsprung's Disease

Hirschsprung's disease is a curious disorder in which the distal part of the bowel, usually the rectum but sometimes the more extensive part

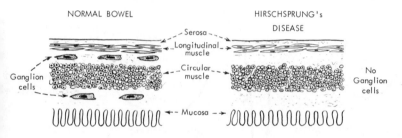

Fig. 21.

extending back into the colon has no ganglion cells in the wall. These ganglion cells are the nerve cells which control the activity of the muscle in the bowel wall. As a result of the lack of these cells the affected part of the bowel does not pass material easily and the baby has an incomplete large bowel obstruction (Fig. 22). Constipation, failure to thrive and abdominal distention are the commonest signs. Operation in infancy is a colostomy performed in the bowel proximal to the aganglionic segment. Care of these infants is similar to that of the baby with imperforate anus and high fistula. If the disease is not diagnosed until childhood rectal washouts may be given daily to clear out the gross accummulation of faecal material from the large bowel. When this has been done and the child's condition is satisfactory laparotomy

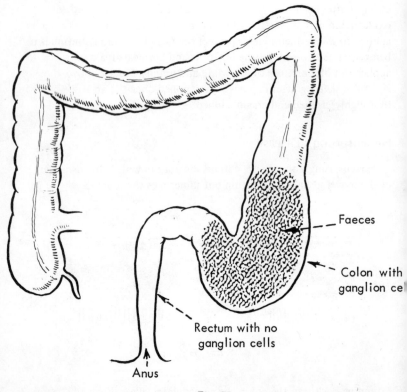

Faeces

Colon with
ganglion ce[ll]

Rectum with no
ganglion cells

Anus

Fig. 22.

is performed and the aganglionic bowel resected. A similar procedure
is done in the infant in whom a colostomy has been performed and
bowel continuity is re-established by one of the operative techniques
e.g. Swenson, du Hamel or Souave.

The post-operative care necessary is similar to that following
laparotomy. If the patient has a colostomy it is closed usually two
weeks after the resection of bowel. When the bowels start moving again
careful attention to the perineal skin and the skin of the buttocks is
necessary for some weeks until the bowels settle down. Long term
results in Hirschsprung's disease are good.

8
Hernia

A hernia is a protrusion or bulge of the viscera from the normal confines of any of the body cavities but herniae from the abdominal cavity are commonest. These herniae are known by the site in which they occur:—

a) inguinal hernia
b) umbilical hernia and exomphalos
c) diaphragmatic hernia

Each of these causes quite a different set of signs and symptoms.

a) Inguinal Hernia and Hydrocele

This is more common in boys than girls and occurs in approximately 2 per cent of the male population. In both sexes during development there is an opening from the abdominal cavity down into the scrotum in the male, or into the labia in the female. In the normal infant this tube of peritoneum closes off leaving the abdominal or peritoneal cavity intact and a small sac of tunica over the testes in the male. However, this tube may fail to close resulting in a hernia into which bowel can prolapse. If there is partial closure leaving a narrow opening which only allows peritoneal fluid to pass down into the scrotum a hydrocele results.

The commonest presentation of an infant or child with an inguinal hernia is for the parents to notice the swelling in the inguinal region which may extend into the scrotum. Sometimes bowel will become stuck in the hernial sac, i.e. an *incarcerated inguinal hernia* and the child will develop colicky abdominal pain and vomiting. If this is allowed to continue for some time the blood supply to the bowel may be cut off and it then becomes a *strangulated hernia.* This dangerous situation is uncommon. The treatment of the child admitted as an emergency with incarcerated hernia is to give him a heavy dose of sedation. Half an hour to one hour later the doctor can then reduce the hernia by gentle compression. The hernia is repaired some days later when swelling has subsided. Rarely the child may have to go to theatre as an emergency to have the incarcerated or strangulated hernia reduced by operation. The pre- and post-operative treatment for such a child is similar to that for a child with intestinal obstruction from any other cause.

Pre-Operative Care

Most children with inguinal herniae are admitted from the waiting list and the routine documentation and care are given. The pre-operative care is simply routine care giving the groins and inguinal region a particularly thorough cleansing prior to operation. At operation the surgeon closes off this abnormal communication from the peritoneal cavity at the inguinal ring. This is done through a small inguinal incision and the wound may be closed with subcuticular sutures which do not need removal, or with interrupted silk sutures.

Post-Operative Care

Post-operative care is routine and the child is allowed home the following day. In some centres this operation (herniotomy) is done in infants and children who are simply admitted as a day case, i.e. admitted in the morning, then operation is performed and the child allowed home later in the day.

Unlike hernia, hydrocele is not a dangerous condition although it is unsightly. The collection of fluid causes considerable scrotal swelling. In the early months of life this is best left as it may cure itself. However, if it is persisting or if the hydrocele is fluctuating indicating there is still a communication with the peritoneal cavity operation similar to that for inguinal hernia is performed.

b) Umbilical Hernia and Exomphalos

Umbilical hernia are common and, although in white races, they are not usually very large, in Negro races they both have a much higher incidence and are of larger size. Umbilical hernia is normal in intra-uterine life at an early age of development. However, the bowel then usually returns into the abdominal cavity as it becomes large enough to accommodate it and the umbilical opening narrows down to a small size so that there are only the blood vessels coming out to the placenta which pass through it

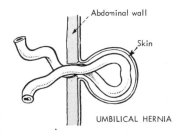

Fig. 23

by birth. When the opening does not close down sufficiently this allows bowel to continue to prolapse from the abdominal cavity. Various degrees of defect are seen. If obvious at birth and there is only a thin covering over the bowel the condition is called exomphalos, but where there is good skin covering the bulge which may become obvious after birth is called an umbilical hernia. With exomphalos the size of the defect may vary considerably in the newborn baby so that with a large exomphalos bowel and liver may prolapse into the sac. These infants are usually operated on very soon after birth and the abdominal wall defect repaired. They require routine care as for any baby having an abdominal operation. Alternatively the thin sac may be painted daily with 2 per cent mercurochrome which hastens growth of skin over the bulge and some years later the hernia is repaired.

The much more common situation is where the baby has apparently returned the gut to the abdominal cavity long before birth but then in the first weeks or months of life a swelling appears in the umbilical region particularly when the baby is straining or crying. This umbilical hernia requires no treatment in the vast majority of white children and in the majority of coloured children. Over the first few years of life the abdominal muscles strengthen and the gap at the umbilicus gradually closes so that at the time of going to school less than 5 per cent of the herniae are still present. If the hernia is still present in the year prior to the child going to school then it is worthwhile repairing it but earlier operation is rarely indicated. The cure rate in coloured children is not quite so

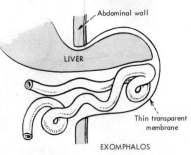

Fig. 24.

high and rather more require operation. Pre- and post-operative care is similar to that described under inguinal hernia except for the babies with exomphalos. These neonates require the routine care of young newborn undergoing operation and slow introduction of feeding in the post-operative period is required as the bowel may be slow in functioning due to the handling at operation. Intravenous fluids are occasionally necessary if the babies cannot take sufficient fluid intake in the first few days of life.

c) Diaphragmatic Hernia

Diaphragmatic hernia is not a very common condition only arising in approximately 1 : 2,000 births, but this can be one of the most acute emergencies in any surgeon's experience. The infant may have difficulty in establishing breathing at birth or in the subsequent few hours develop cardio-respiratory difficulties. The breathing is laboured and the baby either cyanosed or pale ashen grey in appearance. Unless the baby has immediate operation there is little hope of survival. With some infants the diaphragmatic hernia is of smaller size and with these infants and

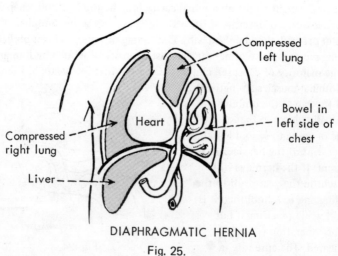

DIAPHRAGMATIC HERNIA
Fig. 25.

children they may survive weeks, months or years before the condition becomes apparent. This is again a defect in the confines of the abdominal cavity where the bowel passes through the diaphragm into the pleural cavity.

Pre-Operative Care

These babies come as an emergency and it is important to have everything ready for treatment of the baby as soon as he is admitted. It is the one condition in which the baby will not infrequently be taken directly to theatre and may already have been intubated and given assisted ventilation before admission. The babies with less severe distress are nursed in a heated incubator in 40 per cent oxygen. The baby is tilted head up (15°) and nursed lying on the side of the hernia.

Post-Operative Care

All of these babies require a special nurse by them until they are over the acute respiratory problems of the immediate post-operative period. With infants over twenty four hours of age careful recording of respiratory rate, pulse or heart rate, and temperature are usually all that is necessary while the baby is nursed in the incubator with increased oxygen (40 per cent). The general condition of the baby is recorded and if he is restless this may be the first signs that he is not getting enough oxygen into the body. The intercostal drain should fluctuate with respiration (see Page 34). Any marked rise in respiratory or pulse rates, in restlessness or in the intercostal drain not oscillating or bubbling off air through the underwaterseal, should be reported.

The infants under 24 hours of age present even greater problems and these may not be able to breathe satisfactorily and so come back from theatre with a nasotracheal tube in position and may be connected to a mechanical ventilator. These infants require the attention described in Chapter 5 for nasotracheal intubation as well as for their intercostal drainage. General nursing care and recording of respiratory rate etc. as described in the previous paragraph are performed by the 'special' nurse. Particular care is taken with the introduction of feeds to these babies as with the increased intra-abdominal tension where there is an increased likelihood of vomiting. Small quantities are given at frequent intervals and the baby gradually worked up on to a normal feeding regime. Chest X-rays of the baby are done to ensure expansion of the lungs is occurring. Once over this severe initial disorder these babies do very well and their long term prognosis, if they survive the first few days of life, is very good indeed.

9
Skin and Subcutaneous Tissue

Haemangioma and Lymphangioma

The skin and subcutaneous tissue not infrequently have abnormalities such as birth marks. These are abnormal collections of blood vessels in the skin and many of them do not require treatment. For instance the so-called strawberry birth marks, i.e. a raised red soft swelling usually appears in the first few weeks of life. It is not usually visible at birth or at most it is a very small spot which grows quite markedly over some months. These are very frightening to the parents. It is important to know that the natural history of these is that they grow for some months, then remain static, and then over the succeeding months or years, gradually fade, ending up as a rather thin area of skin but, provided they have not ulcerated and become infected, the skin is almost normal in character. There is no indication for treatment of them except the few which are growing unusually rapidly or a few which are present in the face. Early treatment of these can stop their further growth. This treatment can be by carbon dioxide snow or by diathermy. In a small baby either of these can be applied without anaesthesia but in the older infant a general anaesthetic is necessary. Routine care is necessary for the child.

Other malformations in the skin may involve lymphatic vessels and these can either take the form of large swellings in the neck, i.e.

cystic hygroma and some of these are so large that they may produce acute respiratory embarrassment and require operation in the immediate post-natal period. The majority are smaller and unsightly. These require a long dissection to excise all the rammifications of these lesions. Routine care is necessary and suction drain may be applied under the flaps of skin to prevent an accummulation of serous fluid in the post-operative period. Other abnormalities of the lymphatic system may be more diffuse and cause widespread subcutaneous swelling. This may affect limbs and give rise to an enormously enlarged limb or may occur on the body wall. These are subject to recurrent attacks of inflammation and are usually treated by surgical excision when the infection has subsided. However, this is not always very successful as there is a marked tendency for recurrence causing an unsightly appearance.

Burns and Scalds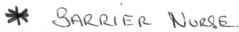

   Damage to the skin by heat is a very common accident in childhood. Where hot water or fluid is spilled the damage is called a scald and with scalds it is usually only the superficial parts of the skin that are damaged. Some of the deeper epithelial elements remain. These will grow out and epithelialise the area, hence skin grafting of scalds does not commonly have to be done. The care of a scalded child differs in this respect from a burned child. However, with burns which can be caused by flame or electric heat the entire thickness of the skin is frequently damaged and for these children as well as the early initial treatment subsequent treatment by skin grafting may be necessary. Emergency treatment of cooling and covering the area with a sterile dressing is usually carried out at home. It is best not to apply any other paste, jam, or other medication. This sterile dressing may be any clean material such as handkerchiefs which have been ironed, cleaned table cloths, etc.

   On admission to hospital the immediate concern is the extent of the scald or burn. If more than 10 per cent of the body surface has been burned the child should have an intravenous infusion established immediately and a regime of intravenous fluids is given amounting to

2 mls. per cent of body area burned per kg. of body weight over the first twenty four hours and half of this volume of fluid should be given in the first eight hours as the loss from the circulation occurs particularly in the first few hours of injury. If there has been a little delay from the time of burning to time of admission it may be difficult to set up an intravenous infusion without doing a cut-down on a vein.

On admission the child will be in distress due to the pain from the scald or burn and sedation should be given. This may be Omnopon 1 mgm per 3 kg. body weight or Pethidine 1 mgm per kg. body weight. The initial dose is given intramuscularly. Initially the scald or burned area can be left exposed placing the child on a sterile sheet in a warm environment with a temperature in the cubicle or isolation area of approximately 25°C. Once the child's circulatory state has been stabilised the area is cleaned and exposed so that a dry coagulum of the exuded plasma is formed over the surface of the raw area. The surgeon may prefer to take the child to theatre, anaesthetise him, clean the area and then dress it i.e. the closed method.

A careful record of the pulse and if it can be taken, the blood pressure is essential over the first forty eight hours after injury. Other observations include an assessment of the peripheral circulation, collection of urine passed, and the general state of the child, whether quiet and restful or distressed, unco-operative and irritable.

Many of these children benefit from Sparine as well as pain killing drugs in the first twenty four hours and antibiotics may be prescribed. Oral fluids are recommended early but given in small quantities at a time. The caloric value of the fluids and diet is stepped up as quickly as possible and it is important to get the maximum nourishment into these children as they have a very high metabolic rate following burning.

Subsequent treatment is to gradually trim off the eschar or dry coagulum as it separates in exposure treatment, or weekly theatre dressings in the closed. If necessary Split skin grafts are taken from the child. Post-operatively these areas are treated either by the exposed or closed methods. The nurse must encourage the child to move his limbs as much as possible to prevent or minimise the development of contractures which may require prolonged physiotherapy and sometimes further surgery.

10
Central Nervous System

Defects in formation of the Central Nervous System are one of the common congenital malformations and occur in Britain in up to five every thousand births. The malformations may be severe, for instance anencephaly where the brain and skull have not formed properly. This defect is inevitably lethal. However, lesser degrees of malformation are common and these are the meningocele and myelomeningocele defects. Spina Bifida (Fig. 26b) may occur without nervous system malformation but it is present in all infants with meningocele group of defects. Hence these malformations are sometimes known collectively as the spina bifida group.

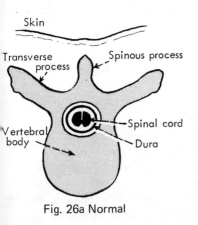

Fig. 26a Normal

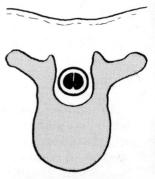

Fig. 26b Spina Bifida

Meningocele (Fig. 26c)

This is a blow-out of the coverings of the spinal cord. It may occur anywhere along the posterior aspect of the spinal cord or over the brain but the commonest sites are the lumbar and occipital regions. With this defect there is no paralysis below the level of the meningocele as the actual nerves are not involved but only the covering membranes.

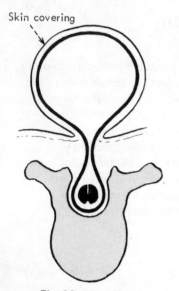

Skin covering

Fig. 26c Meningocele

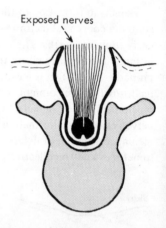

Exposed nerves

Fig. 26d Myelomeningocele

Myelomeningocele (Fig. 26d)

This is a more severe form of the same type of defect where not only is there a blow-out of the coverings but the nerves come out to the surface. Inevitably with this defect there is some paralysis which may be fairly minor with only a few muscle groups affected or it may be more severe and affect all muscles to the lower limbs and the nerve supply to and from the bladder and large bowel. These defects are obvious at birth and in the last ten years the standard form of treatment has been that they are operated on immediately after birth to minimise the paralysis and when the spinal cord is covered again the danger of ascending infection is eliminated. The defective nerve supply affects the sensory side as well as the motor so that the feet and lower limbs of these babies must be handled with care. Manipulations must be done carefully and any splints applied must be padded or very chronic pressure sores develop. They also need gentle handling as the bones are often more fragile than normal and fracture easily with minimal trauma.

Hydrocephalus

This is where there is an increase in the quantity of fluid retained inside the brain causing enlargement of the skull. In the normal individual cerebro-spinal fluid is formed in the ventricles, passed from the lateral ventricles to third ventricle, down to fourth ventricle, and then out over the surface of the brain and the spinal cord. Frequently in children with Myelomeningocele there is a defect of this circulation so that cerebrospinal fluid cannot escape from inside the brain and this causes progressive expansion of the ventricles and therefore expansion of the brain and of the head. Also following meningitis and sometimes for other more obscure reasons the outflow of cerebrospinal fluid from the ventricles is blocked and hydrocephalus then develops. Babies suspected of having hydrocephalus or infants with myelomeningocele have their head circumference measured by passing a tape around the occiput, round the skull over the most prominent part of the frontal bone and recording the size. This is then charted against the normal head circumference of an infant of that age. Serial readings are made and

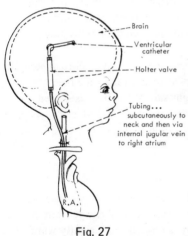

Brain

Ventricular catheter

Holter valve

Tubing...
subcutaneously to
neck and then via
internal jugular vein
to right atrium

R.A.

Fig. 27

63

if the rate of the skull growth is greater than the normal increase in skull circumference which occurs in the first weeks and months of life, then progressive hydrocephalus is developing. For this, drainage of the cerebrospinal fluid from the lateral ventricle through a one way valve system such as the Holter, Dahl-Wade, or Pudenz valves is used and a distal catheter from the valve passes down into the jugular vein and the right side of the heart. In half the children with such a drainage system it continues to work satisfactorily over the years, but in the remaining half further operation may become necessary.

Pre-Operative Care

The neonate with a myelomeningolece is usually operated on during the first day of life. The exposed nervous tissue is protected by a sterile dressing which has been soaked in normal saline. The back is X-rayed and a careful muscle chart record is made on the muscle groups functioning before operation. The baby is given Vitamin K and premedication.

The infant with hydrocephalus has a specimen of cerebrospinal fluid sent for culture and one for chemical analysis at the time the ventriculogram is performed. The right side of the head is shaved and washed with betadine the night before operation. Blood is grouped and cross-matched and the infants haemoglobin is checked.

Post-Operative Care

The baby, following closure of the back, usually settles quickly and commences feeding four hours later. These infants' temperature is often very labile and falls easily if the baby is not kept sufficiently warm. The lower limbs are put through a full range of movements daily and manipulation of any deformed joints is carried out. The baby's abdomen is felt before each feed and if the bladder is not emptying spontaneously it is expressed. Longer term problems are:-

1 Hydrocephalus which may develop.
2 Orthopaedic problems related to paralysed groups of muscles.

3 Urological problems due to interference with the normal bladder innervation.

In post-operative nursing of the hydrocephalic infant who has a drainage procedure routine care is necessary. If too much cerebrospinal fluid is draining in the early stages, the fontanelles become sunken. A 15° head down tilt results in a decrease in drainage of cerebrospinal fluid and in a few days the baby can be nursed lying flat again. If the valve subsequently blocks the signs are:-

a) Increasing head size
b) Increased prominence of veins over the scalp
c) Vomiting and irritability
d) Slow pulse
e) Loss of consciousness
f) Respiratory arrest may occur suddenly

Revision of the valve is necessary whenever it is clear that it is not functioning and the head size is increasing or the infant or child has raised intracranial pressure.

The urological problem can be anticipated and it is worth doing an intravenous pyelogram on the baby's first admission. Some will already be abnormal. Specimens of urine have to be examined regularly and urinary diversion may later become necessary (Page 72).

Tumour

Tumours arising in the central nervous system may cause headache, vomiting, nausea, irritability, loss of balance or loss of consciousness. These are investigated by ventriculogram and arteriogram and treated by surgery and radiotherapy.

Trauma to the Head

This is very common in infants and children. Most toddlers when starting to crawl and walk receive bumps to the head which do them no harm. A bruise or haematoma may develop but once the child has been comforted all is forgotten until the next time. Older children, however, are more adventurous and as a result may fall from a height or be knocked down by an automobile. Patients admitted as an emergency with head injuries can be divided into three categories:-

a) Those who may be unconscious for a few minutes following the accident and have minor lacerations or cranial fractures of the vault of the skull without a break in the skin. They recover very quickly and after treatment of any superficial wounds, bed rest and observation for twenty four hours can be allowed home.

b) With more serious injury and usually with a more prolonged loss of consciousness, careful observation is necessary and they may be detained for longer.

c) Severe injury, i.e. those with a fractured base of skull or extensive intracerebral injury and those patients may have permanent brain damage.

Treatment of patients with head injuries varies with the extent of injury. Where the child is conscious on admission but drowsy a close watch must be kept on his condition and any twitching, change in colour, or laboured breathing reported. The *following vital signs should always be observed* and written into the report:—

a) *Clear airway* must be maintained. In the deeply unconscious insertion of an oral airway, endotracheal tube or tracheostomy may be necessary.

b) *Level of consciousness.* Is the child:-
   1 Fully conscious and alert
   2 Drowsy but responding to stimuli
   3 Deeply unconscious and not responding

c) *Pulse and respiratory rates and blood pressure* should be done half hourly or more frequently if the doctor requests. A fall in pulse rate or alteration in blood pressure may indicate internal haemorrhage and increased intracranial pressure.

d) *Re-action of pupils to light* and if the pupils are equal. Dilated or unequal pupils may indicate intracranial bleeding point.

e) *Tone in the limb muscles* and ability to move all limbs.

When the nurse is notified of a patient to be admitted due to a head injury a bed or a cot should be prepared for the child. A bed elevator should be at hand and if multiple injuries are present resuscitation should be available. This should consist of:—

> Airway or endotracheal tube
> Laryngoscope and blade
> Suction catheters
> Connections for catheters and tubing
> Lubricant (K—Y jelly)
> Suction
> Adhesive tape
> Oxygen supply
> Face mask

If the child is conscious he should be nursed flat. Fluids are usually restricted for the first few hours if the child has been vomiting but should be introduced thereafter and gradually increased. Light diet may be given the following day when the child is recovering.

Where the child is unconscious on admission the vital signs are recorded and any change reported immediately to doctor. An adequate airway must always be maintained. Fluids may have to be given intravenously, e.g. plasma or blood if the child is shocked or manitol for cerebral oedema. A rise of temperature should be reported and the child kept cool either by tepid sponging or blowing a cool stream of air over the exposed child. Oral hygiene should be attended to at least four hourly and care given to pressure areas. Use of a ripple bed may be made. With this, pressure is not continuously on one area and danger of skin necrosis is minimised. The child's position should be changed hourly, gradually extending the interval to four hourly. If unconsciousness continues beyond twenty four hours tube feeding becomes necessary.

11
Genito-Urinary Tract

Indications for operation on the genito-urinary tract in infants and children are:—

a) Malformations, e.g. cystic kidney and hypospadias
b) Tumours, e.g. nephroblastoma
c) Obstruction to urine flow, e.g. urethral valves
d) Recurrent infection, and
e) Abnormalities of the genital organs, e.g. undescended testis

The urinary tract in the normal child consists of two kidneys lying high in the posterior abdominal wall through which urine passes into the pelvis of the kidney along the ureters to the bladder. Urine is retained in the bladder until there is sufficient quantity and then it is passed along the urethra to the exterior. Micurition, i.e. passing urine, is a reflex in the young infant but gradually the child becomes able to control when he will empty his bladder. Some children are much slower in the ability to control their bladder particularly at night. Many children may continue to bed wet long after they have gone to school but settle in time.

a) Malformations

Various forms of cystic disease of the kidneys may occur. With multi-cystic kidney there is a large abdominal mass which is often detected in the neonatal period. In this condition the kidney on the affected side is replaced by cysts and investigation by intravenous pyelogram shows no renal function on that side. Lower in the urinary tract malformations such as ectopia vesicae, i.e. where the bladder has not closed properly and is lying open in the lower part of the abdominal wall are obvious at birth. Urine drains from the ureters on to the surface. The condition is not usually treated in the neonatal period but once the child is approximately one year old attempt at reconstruction of the bladder is performed. These children may ultimately require urinary diversion, i.e. where the ureters are led into an isolated loop of bowel from which the urine drains on to the surface of the abdominal wall where it can be collected in a bag applied to the abdomen. Less severe malformations occur, for instance the hypospadias, where the opening of the urethra is not on the tip of the penis but is along the under surface. This is discussed on page 74.

b) Tumours

The kidney is one of the commoner sites of malignant tumour in children. This usually becomes apparent as a large abdominal mass in a child who has vague abdominal pain or discomfort, vomiting or diarrhoea. Removal of the kidney followed by radiotherapy and courses of intravenous Actinomycin D result in half of these children surviving. The remainder develop progressive disease which ultimately proves fatal.

c) Obstruction to Urine Flow

In a urinary tract which has a congenital abnormality it is more susceptible to infection than the normal and particularly where the abnormality causes hold-up of urine infection can be dangerous. The commoner sites for obstruction are at the junction of the pelvis and the ureter causing hydronephrosis or at the junction of ureter and bladder causing hydronephrosis and hydro-ureter, or at the bladder neck and posterior urethra where both kidneys, ureters and also the bladder are affected. Surgical treatment can usually relieve the obstruction.

d) Recurrent Infection

This may be superimposed on a malformation or it may occur in a child where the normal one way passage of urine from ureters into bladder is upset so that urine can easily reflux from bladder into ureters. The infection causes pyrexia, general malaise and frequently vomiting as well as discomfort in passing urine and increased frequency in passing it.

e) Genital Abnormalities

Operation on the genital tract in the male is usually on the testes. A common abnormality is that the testes do not settle in the normal scrotal position. They may fail to descend from the abdominal cavity into the scrotum or in descent they may move in the wrong direction. Unless the testis is placed in the scrotum it will not function normally. This and other genital abnormalities are discussed after the special post-operative care following urinary tract operations.

Pre-Operative Care

General care is the same for children undergoing urinary tract surgery as for those with any other abdominal procedure. Careful fluid intake and output charts should be maintained.

Post-Operative Care

This varies with the operation performed. Frequently tubes draining urine are left in either at kidney level (nephrostomy), into bladder (cystostomy) or along the urethra into the bladder, and these must be kept in situ particularly in the first few days after operation. It is very important that these are not displaced as it may be difficult at this point to replace them. Nephrostomy and cystostomy tubes are usually strapped with adhesive strapping to the body wall. It is rather more difficult to fix a transurethral catheter in a child. As well as the above, drainage of urine may be performed through ureterostomies, i.e. where a loop of ureter is brought out similar to that done in performing colostomy and this loop of ureter is opened so that urine can freely discharge on to the anterior abdominal wall. These various methods of draining urine require special care post-operatively.

Nephrostomy

On return from theatre the child who has had a nephrostomy performed will have the tube firmly strapped to the skin in the loin and usually the nephrostomy catheter is spigotted at this time. The

70

ward nurse has then to connect this to a urine collecting bag which is hung by the bedside. There are bags available which have markings on the side which indicate the volume of urine in the bag when it is hanging vertically. From this bag there is a tube with a connector piece on the end of it. This connector is joined into the nephrostomy tube and the junction strapped. Urine can then drain freely from the kidney along the nephrostomy tube and into the collecting bag. The collecting bag is hung from the side of the bed but once the child is sufficiently recovered this may be suspended from his waist and the child may be up and running around the ward although he has nephrostomies. Continuous drainage is maintained while nephrostomies are in situ. The skin around the entrance of the nephrostomy tube is cleaned with saline and hibitane solution and the tube firmly restrapped in position. When the nephrostomy tube has to be removed the strapping is taken off, the area around cleaned and the tube simply pulled out. A sterile dressing is then applied over the opening and usually this closes within forty-eight hours.

Ureterostomy

As ureterostomies continuously discharge urine on to the abdominal wall the skin tends to become macerated and excoriated. Care of the skin is similar to that necessary for the baby or child with colostomy and as with colostomy in the small child no appliance is usually fitted to the abdominal wall, whereas in the older child with ureterostomy a collecting apparatus may be applied to the anterior abdominal wall. This is similar to that for an ileostomy (Figs. 18 and 19).

Cystostomy

This is usually done as a temporary procedure following operations on the bladder. The catheter is connected to drainage bag as described for nephrostomy and after some days the tube may be spigoted off intermittently and the child allowed up. This is seldom used for prolonged drainage. Care of the skin around the catheter is similar to the nephrostomy tube.

Urinary Diversion

The commonest urinary diversion is to use a loop of ileum but alternatively a loop of colon may be used or sometimes the grossly enlarged ureters are brought on to the skin surface as the stoma. This is a major procedure and the child on return from theatre will have an intravenous infusion running and this has to be maintained. A nasogastric tube may be in position and this will require four hourly aspiration. The loop of ileum brought out on the anterior abdominal wall usually has a urine bag applied over it and a catheter inserted into this so that urine can be aspirated every two hours and the volume

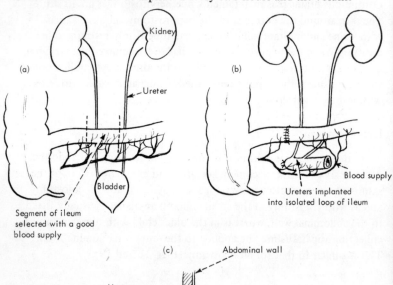

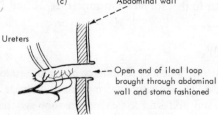

Fig. 28 Urinary Diversion

passed recorded. There may be a drain into the peritoneal cavity and this requires shortening after forty-eight hours and removal after this. It is important that the ileal stoma is not covered in the post-operative period as the blood supply to this can become impaired and then the colour of the bowel deteriorates and it becomes bluish. This may necessitate re-operation. Once the abdominal wall is healed and the stitches are removed after ten days the surgical appliance officer will fit an appliance similar to that for a colostomy except for the bag fitted over the ileal loop has a tap on it which allows frequent emptying of the urine without removal of the apparatus. Depending on the volume of urine passed the bag is emptied either two hourly or at less frequent intervals. This is simply done by turning the tap and draining urine into a receptacle.

The skin around the ileostomy may give trouble as with colostomy. However, if a good stoma has been made by the surgeon and a satisfactory appliance is put on the child little trouble is experienced. The period of time which the appliance will remain stuck to the abdominal wall varies and when it is becoming loose then it is removed, the skin cleaned and the stoma washed with soap and water and thoroughly dried. The plaster is removed with Zoff and then the procedure described for sticking a colostomy bag is repeated, applying the collecting apparatus over the ileal loop. This may not require to be changed for a further week but the urine collecting bag has to be removed from the phlange daily and this is thoroughly washed, alternatively disposable bags are used. As these children usually have damaged urinary tracts antibiotic therapy is necessary and is continued for some time after operation. Within two or three days of operation they are back on light diet and they are allowed up. Within a week of operation children are usually moving around freely whereas adults are still very conscious of a recent operation. Before discharge of the child the parents are instructed in the care of the stoma and application of the bags. The child is seen soon after discharge to ensure the parents and child are managing satisfactorily.

The Genital Organs

In the male the testes and penis commonly require operation

whereas in the female child operation on the genital tract is uncommon.

Testes

The testes develop in the abdomen and move down into the scrotum before birth. This descent of the testes may be arrested, i.e. undescended testis, or the testis may not descend along the correct line, i.e. ectopic testis. These can be diagnosed in the neonatal period but more commonly are noted at routine school medical examinations. If the testes are allowed to remain in a high abnormal position they do not develop their function of producing sperm satisfactorily and so operation (orchidopexy) is advised to try and bring them into a normal position in the scrotum.

The child admitted for orchidopexy has routine pre-operative care. Post-operative care is routine and these children may require sedation as they are often in discomfort. After their stitches are removed they are allowed home but should not indulge in violet physical activity for a month after operation.

Hypospadias

Hypospadias is where the terminal urethral oriface opens somewhere along the shaft of the penis, or in the perineum. The prepuce may appear 'hooded' and the penis may be curved. Pre-operatively no special treatment is required. Post-operatively the child usually has a urethral catheter, or a catheter inserted behind the scrotum to the bladder (perineal urethrostomy) which remains in position for five to ten days. Antibiotics are given while the catheter is in situ. The catheter is connected to a urine drainage bag which is attached to the cot or bed. The child should be encouraged to drink plenty of fluids. When the catheter is removed the child finds it easier to pass urine while in a warm Sitz bath (salt and water) on the first one or two occasions. At operation the skin on the dorsum of the penis is divided to relieve tension on the suture line. The wound is kept clean and dry. The raw area heals in ten—fourteen days.

Fused Labiae

This uncommon condition in little girls is where the labiae are fused. This is simply the adhesion between the labia and there is usually sufficient opening anteriorly for the child to be able to pass urine satisfactorily. This is a perfectly simple condition and, if seen in the neonate, gentle pressure on either side will split the labiae and expose a normal vaginal oriface. In the older child a brief general anaesthetic is necessary as it is painful separating the labia. After separation of the labia the area is liberally smeared with Vaseline to prevent re-adhesion and this is repeated after each micturition or nappie change for a week. No long term difficulties arise from this condition.

Imperforate Hymen

With imperforate hymen the female child either presents at birth with a cystic swelling bulging from the perineum between the labia and some times with a large mass in the lower part of the abdomen. In extreme cases this swelling of the vagina may cause pressure on the ureters and cause bilateral hydronephrosis and hydro-ureter. The distended vagina is filled by secretions from the baby's uterus. This does not occur in all cases of imperforate hymen and some may not collect sufficient material for presentation to occur at this age. In these cases the condition is not detected until puberty and then the girl fails to menstruate. Her menstrual flow, in fact, is obstructed by the imperforate hymen and will give abdominal pain at the time of each menstrual cycle. On examination soon after puberty, the distended vagina will be detected. Operation may be a small perineal procedure or a large combined abdominal and perineal approach.

Inter-Sex

In the first weeks of pregnancy the baby developing in utero has the ability to develop into either sex. However, about the fourth month the change into female or male occurs depending on the chromosome contents of the baby's cells. The female baby has forty-four plus two X chromosomes, while the male has forty-four chromosomes plus an X and a Y chromosome. In a very few children this clear differentiation into female or male may not occur. These children present complex problems. When such a baby is born the external genitalia will not be characteristic of the male child or of the female child. It is very important then that this very perplexing situation should be explained to the parents and that the baby should not be registered as male or female until the doctors have done various investigations and examinations to determine the true sex of the child or to determine what sex it is best to rear the child as. There are various causes of ambiguous genitalia.

12
Hospital Discharge

Discharging a patient from hospital can be a very happy day for nursing staff, parents and child. The parents, who may be having their child home perhaps after a lengthy illness, or even looking forward to having the new baby home, are very often excited and overjoyed and if given verbal instructions on dates for return may easily forget them. Hence dates and time of follow-up appointment, and any important instructions, should be given in writing.

Where a baby is going home for the first time it is important to have the mother come and care for the infant for a day or two prior to discharge. If possible she should live in and care for the baby so that when the sister is happy that the mother can cope and the doctors think the baby fit he can go home safely. The nurse first performs the procedures with the mother present then next time supervises mother in the procedure, this being done until the mother has confidence in handling the infant.

In the case of the infant or child having had a colostomy, ileostomy, gastrostomy or some form of splinting performed, then the mother and the child, if old enough, should be instructed and must practise the special care necessary until they are quite sure of it. For instance, with colostomy the parents, usually more so than the child, may become very upset on at first seeing it. To them the area looks very raw and sore and the mother may feel she cannot touch it for fear of hurting her child. The nurse should prepare the parents before showing them the affected area, reminding them that feelings of disgust and horror can be transmitted to the older child through the expression on their faces.

Instructions when possible should always be written for the parents, making sure that they have been understood. It is also important to make sure they are practical, e.g. it is no use saying 'continue giving sitz baths' when

a) there is no bath at home,
b) they do not understand 'sitz.'

What should be said is that the affected area be immersed in salted warm water be it in a bath, sink or basin.

Help from the Medical Social Worker may be necessary on account of emotional, financial, or physical difficulties in the home. If brought early enough into the discussions on the patient these problems may all be alleviated before the child goes home or at least a start to organising suitable housing, for instance, for a child with severe physical handicap may be started. The family may require continued support from the Medical Social Worker and this may save unnecessary hospitalisation of the child on future occasions.

If the child is to continue on treatment at home it is essential that the parents are given a sufficient supply of medicine to last until their general practitioner has had full details from the hospital so that he can repeat the prescriptions for further supplies if necessary. The parents should also know that if in trouble they may phone for advice.

Index

Throughout this book correct medical terms have been used—and where possible explained. Do not hesitate to ask when you do not understand the meaning of a word or procedure. Every nurse once knew as much as you—yet see what she seems to know now.

Learn to use medical terms correctly and you will find that this increases your efficiency and your confidence in yourself.

Wilm's Tumour. see page 43.

NOTES

NOTES

NOTES

NOTES

NOTES

NOTES

NOTES

NOTES